Vortex of Feelings: The Early Months

Book II

The Psychological Survival Guide for Parents

by

Dr. Paul Peebles

Best Read Before Delivery

(although there is no expiration date)

OMG! We're Pregnant is the beginning book of *The Psychological Survival Guide for Parents* landmark series. It deals mainly with the psychological development of parents during pregnancy and delivery, and delves further into the psyche of the newborn.

This book, *Vortex of Feelings: The Early Months,* is the second in the series. Its concerns are regarding parents' relationships with each other, their child, and others during primarily the early months. Thus, this ultimate rite of passage continues to flourish even after delivery.

Book III, soon to arrive, unmasks life's greatest recurrent fear: Separation Fear(s), or *"Don't Leave Me!"*

Other Books to come.

Published by
Pediatric Care Publications, LLC
Haverford, PA, USA

Photographs by parents and by Karin Kristine Ottesen,
Paul Peebles, Amanda Dickson, and Lisa Helfer
Cartoons by Sari Werner & Rose Jaffe
Graphics by Rose Jaffe
Collage Graphics by Joe Mach
Interior Book Design by Darlene Swanson

Library of Congress Control Number: 2017937583
Peebles, Paul
Vortex of Feelings: The Early Months / by Paul Peebles, MD
Book II, The Psychological Survival Guide for Parents

1. Family 2. Child Care 3. Pregnancy 4. Childbirth
5. Parenting 6. Relationships 7. Life Cycle Human
8. Prenatal Care 9. Early Childhood 10. Psychology 11. Postnatal Care
12. Child Health 13. Sociology 14. Child Development 15. Marriage 16. Divorce

includes index and glossary
includes illustrations
ISBN-13: 978-0-9970762-3-3
ISBN-10: 0-9970762-3-2

Printed in the United States of America
www.drpaulpeebles.com
@drpaulpeebles
/drpaulpeebles

Thank You

Amazing thanks to Dr. Fred Lovejoy for some wonderful and extraordinarily thoughtful editing and guidance.

Special thanks to my sister Mary Jo Peebles, PhD, for great discussion and contributions as a reviewer/editor with her expertise in Child and Adult Psychology and Psychoanalysis.

A very big thanks to Michelle Beckett for wonderful copy-editing... and, great contributions!

I owe a great debt to Kendra Rubinfeld and Travis Hare for not just PR but for their amazing supportive navigation.

My deepest thanks to my wife Inger, my daughter Rebecka, my son Gustav, my daughter-in-law Amanda Pollak, and my son-in-law Todd Ridky for ever-present support with advice and insights.

And, very importantly, thanks to the parents who permitted photos of themselves and/or their children.

To Those Who Wrote This Series

Many people have contributed to the ideas put forth in these books. I humbly thank them.

However, some very special thanks belong to all my patients, both the children and their parents. It is they who have given me the essence of this book(s). Indeed, they have written this series. It is about their concerns. I want to thank them for having shared their lives with me over the years. They have taught me a lot, and they have made this book and its series possible. As many an author has said, the words in this book(s) are not from me but through me.

Thank You

Dedication

To Parents:

If we can grow with our children,
is that not better for all?

Table of Contents

Part I: The Initial Vortex

Part II: Does He Recognize Me?

Part III: Other Actors in This Rite of Passage

Part IV: Out of the Swirling Fog

List of Anecdotes

Note Regarding Terminology

Today's parents are m/f, m/m, f/f, or single. So, in writing herein and in the rest of the series, *here's how it goes:* "Mother" is the title for the one with the mothering role. That can be a wife as well, and it can be an adopting mother, or a spouse in the mothering role in the f/f relationship, or a single mother. "Father" is used for the one in the fathering role, even in the m/m relationship. These roles, while they may be **gender related**, are **not gender specific**. They are also not determined by the allocation of the usual labor efforts required in child rearing and maintaining the nest, such as men taking care of exterior spaces of the house and women taking care of the interior. These are "parenting roles." What is observed is that one parent takes on the mothering role and the other takes on the fathering role, regardless of whether it is a m/f, m/m, or f/f relationship. A single mother or father takes on both roles. Clearly, breastfeeding issues do not apply to the f/f relationship, but the Intruder Complex does. So not every issue described in this series will apply to every parent.

But it is nice for us to learn what others are experiencing. We can then support each other.

This series investigates and concentrates on ***relationships***. It does not look at just parent and child but particularly focuses on the actual relationships between parents, as partners, or between a single parent and his/her sense of self as now both m/f. These relationships begin when parents couple, and readjust when a child comes on the scene. The series also observes (dissects) the resultant stresses that inevitably ripple through all those relationships as the family emerges. The series probes further scrutinizing the relationships and stresses also originating from others outside of the core family.

It is a Modern Guide for the Modern Family. This is 21st-Century Parenting.

We are all parents,
and we all have
our children in common.

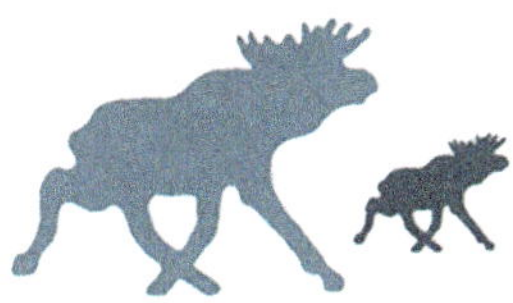

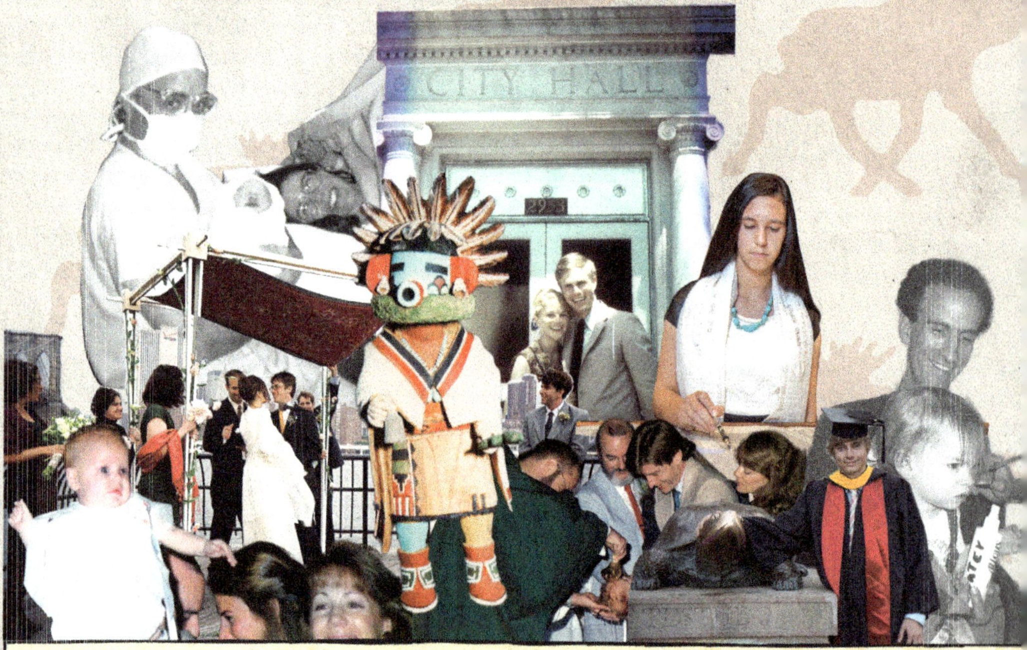

RITES OF PASSAGE

Prequel:
A Rite of Passage

"I didn't grow up until I had a kid."
—Billy Joel, 1990

A Reality Tale

The reality tale spun initially in *OMG! We're Pregnant* continues herein. This tale weaves a mosaic with threads from the anthropology of rites and rituals, the psychodynamic theory of attachment and its pursuant separation fears, the psychology of "ghosts in the nursery," success neurosis, and much more. It offers practical and successful coping concepts from the experience of parents and modern pediatric medicine.

It is about
the Varieties of Parental Experiences.

Whereas *OMG! We're Pregnant* discusses these concepts during pregnancy and delivery, this book covers the amazing and hugely consuming vortex of the first months that follow birth.

Marriage, the Penultimate Step

Marriage is the **penultimate** step for men and women into adulthood. Having a child is the **ultimate** rite of passage required to emerge as adults fulfilled, accomplished, and standing as independent beings. Some may disagree with these statements but I would argue that these are the tenets, the operating codes, of our current society and most other cultures, whether we wish it to be the case or not.

The Ultimate Step

Having a child is indeed a rite of passage, even more so than a confirmation, bar mitzvah, college graduation, or marriage. That fact alone explains a great deal about the behavior of parents-to-be and those around them. As Billy Joel starkly stated, *"I didn't grow up until I had a kid."*

For those going through it, as in all rites of passage, it is important for it to appear as if it were their accomplishment. Parents want control—they want to do as much as they can for themselves so that they, and others, will view them as successful adults to be admired and celebrated by relatives and friends.

While parents grow up, others react. Some are supportive and respectful, while others behave almost enviously, insisting that new parents suffer through this rite of passage as if they were pledging a sorority or fraternity.

Conflicts for Parents

Some assume that perhaps only aging transpires once physical adulthood is attained. Yet having a child and helping him mature and blossom can bring about a completely new insight into and rejuvenating perception of oneself. This maturation of parents presents an opportunity to grow further personally, and to alter goals and priorities in life. And, this continued emotional growth and maturity can be the source of some wonderful satisfaction. A chance to truly define one's self.

But the process is complicated and difficult for many reasons. While children may be longed for and cherished, they profoundly intrude into the intimacy we have developed with our spouse/partner. Enter The Intruder Complex. On top of that, other conflicts arise from temperament issues, attachment and separation conflicts, and "Ghosts in the Nursery," just to mention a few.

The following tale for introduction is not a conglomerate and the actors on the stage are not amalgams, as in most other anecdotes in this series. Harry's mother has told her story in its entirety and, with her permission, it is printed herein in her very words.

It illustrates many of the themes and conflicts mentioned above, and others that follow later in this book: love and worry, success and failure, the grading system, the effect of friends and family, everyone's advice, the effect of the parents' own childhoods on their parenting, the mother's feeling of self-importance, the need to be perfect, and the worry: *"I feel like I am being constantly evaluated."*

Discussions follow, and these themes will be dissected later as this book and its sequels unfold:

Trying to Please Everyone, but Not Harry

> ***At three days of age:*** *"Harry wouldn't latch on to the right side [breast] at all at home. I was significantly engorged since yesterday when the milk came in, especially on the right side. My nipples were slightly sore but I was very worried about the problem on the right side. There was some jaundice but they said it wasn't bad. Since the right side was engorged, the lactation consultant told me to, before breast-feeding, pump on that side to soften it to help the latching on. I was instructed to keep a log of input and output. They told me to breast-feed 8–18 times per day with a minimum of 10–15 minutes per side."*
>
> ***At two weeks:*** *"I called a doula. She came to my house and basically gave me the same advice. I started pumping to relieve the engorgement in order to allow him to attach. But then I gave breast milk via bottle. He was awake and ravenous during the day. But with giving either formula or breast milk via bottle, he started to sleep at night. They asked me about urine and stool, 'That's going fine.'"*

At three weeks: *"I am really worried about this breast-feeding. He wants to feed all the time, especially between 6 p.m. and 11 p.m. He wants way more than 10 minutes per side. So, I've given him the bottle, around 3 ounces around three times at night. He feeds well and sleeps well when I do that. My husband and I feel like this breast-feeding is just too much. It does not allow for any other daily activities. But I want to keep trying; I'm told it is really good for the baby."*

At one month: *"I began giving more and more formula, he takes 3 ounces out of six. I spent an hour talking with the lactation consultant about increasing the day and evening frequency to increase the milk flow. This did not feel right. I am sure that I did not look satisfied but I said, 'I'll try it.' I agreed to sit and talk with her for an hour or so in a week from now. As she left I sort of said, 'I'll try it.'"*

Thirteen days later (~1.5 months of age): *"Well, he's on formula and I feel much better. We have had constant visitors since his birth. They all came in with advice and criticism. I feel like I am being constantly evaluated. I feel like I have to meet certain standards: my own family's, my husband's, his family's, and our friends'. I want to satisfy them and make them happy; but my instincts as a mother are out the door. My mom is the biggest influence. Everything for her is a major chore and she's the victim of all these problems. But what is crazy is that if something is working out and it's enjoyable, then she feels that something is wrong. Do you believe that? On top of that my father is a perfectionist with very high expectations. And I'll never reach those expectations. I don't want one more person coming in telling me what to do. I myself need to figure out what to do to become a good mother."*

One week later (close to two months of age): *"My husband is great. He gives me a lot of leeway on what to do. He leaves it to* *me. My brother is here now. He doesn't know anything about babies. But he always thinks he's right. He sure puts me in a nervous state. His love life is a mess, and it's like I'm his mom. But it puts pressure on me to recommend decisions for him."*

"I'm afraid [Harry] won't love me. He's just started to smile and smiles more at his father. I think I know where I'm heading, but I have got to break through the fear of advice and rejection, especially the rejection from Harry. My husband is soothing; he and Harry listen to music together. I do all of the care giving, the feeding, and the diaper changes. My husband when he comes home from work gets all the cream. He got the first and for a while the only smile. I was really jealous. When I finally got my first smile, I melted."

"I'm already thinking that the second will be easier."

I, the pediatrician, asked about her background:
"Up until 10 to 11 years of age, I was always homesick. At 11 [years of age], the Girl Scouts helped me and I enjoyed it. I felt freer when I knew I was OK by myself. My parents had three children, I was the youngest... the baby who could do no wrong. My mother always held onto me. My brother and my sister were always into trouble. My sister always thought she wasn't wanted. I always thought it was important to do well in school and to stay away from drugs. I got my praise by being good. I went away, I was the first one to go to college. I was the first to get an MBA. My brother and sister are still trying to catch up. All of us were competing for my parents' approval, and my parents think that what I do is better. My parents keep enabling my brother. I was the last to leave home. I am the peacemaker in the family. I have to keep everyone together. I shine by being so good. My mother and father are not emotion-oriented. My dad is not a family-type dad; he's more interested

in his career. Even at Christmastime everyone expects me to be the one to give out the presents under the tree."

"My husband is supporting me and says I'm a great mom. But I'm always worried that I'm not doing enough. Am I hurting Harry by giving into all of his needs? Sometimes he gets bored, and I feel I must entertain him. Already, I'm too tough on myself."

This mother felt her own parents were emotionally unavailable as she grew up (see Ghosts in the Nursery). She was trying to replace this emotional loss from her own childhood by doing what she could to keep both her own and her parents' families intact, even sacrificing breast-feeding for the sake of others' happiness.

More recently: *"By the way, I'm pregnant and my husband and I have already told everyone that we want no visitors until after a few months [of age]. I want to breast-feed this second child."*

Ultimately, she realized that taking on the idealized, self-important role of the hub of the family was negatively impacting Harry. She gave up the need to be needed and the need to be perfect; and Harry thrived and the parents were happy.

Again, this mother's anecdote illustrates many themes and conflicts. These themes will be brought to light, and dissected as this book and its sequels unfold.

Part I:
The Initial VORTEX

"The first six weeks were the worst weeks of my entire life!"

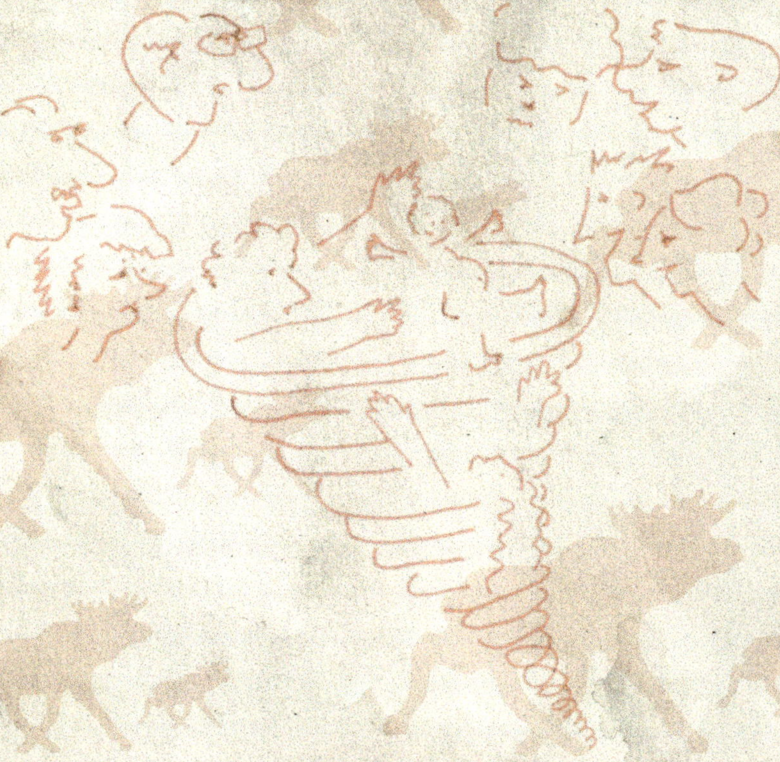

Chapter I:
What Drives the Whirlwinds?

Powerful feelings, during pregnancy, at birth, and after the infant is born, are evoked from the crisis of change, the thrill and worry of accomplishment, and the extraordinary challenge to parental intimacy. Concern and fears abound: *"Am I ready for the overwhelming responsibility of a dependent child?"* Indeed, the first six weeks are often described as *"the worst weeks of my entire life."* At the same time, parents develop an intense intimacy with their new infant. Throwing "The Intruder Complex" into this mixture of joy and sadness can further create a sense of being overwhelmed and confused. To manage our feelings, we must sort them out. To do that we will go from the obvious whirlwinds to the sideswiping gusts that make up this vortex during the first months after the baby's arrival. As parents swim out of the vortex they may not even realize how tough these first weeks are until they are beyond these foggy first days and weeks and look back on their experiences.

Delivery

"It is the best of times, it is the worst of times."

It is miraculous to see this little one emerge. Often, the only words that come close to expressing the awe are, *"I can't believe he's mine."* While worries and any deviations from what was expected compete with that elation, the joy truly takes over during these special moments.

Exhaustion

But then the early weeks become utterly exhausting. Lack of sleep, decreasing tolerance to frustration, promotes irritability. Parents often ask, *"When will he sleep through the night?"* which really means, *"When will I get some sleep?"*

Besides surviving the after-effects of labor, delivery, and the ensuing hormonal changes, parents are awake several times a night (especially those breast-feeding), not only for feedings but also to fearfully observe the sleeping infant. The sleep parents escape to snatch happens only in bits and pieces, which are far from restful. And then the demands of daytime (work, chores) prevent most parents from catching up on the sleep.

Seesaw Emotions

The Confusion of Joy and Sadness

Along with the thrill of this infant's arrival, conflict and confusion occur when joy and sadness mix: This bundle of a baby paints a new look on parents' lives. This new arrival adds purpose, joy, and a sense of fulfillment. He needs to be held and responds to comfort and nourishment. Additionally, the rite of passage (having a child) is over. All the relatives and friends have rejoiced, as have the parents. Unconditional love emerges... but also brings worries and vulnerabilities. The bottom-line is blessed, and cursed by the axiom: **Once you love, you worry.** So, there are losses. But they are far and away offset by the gains.

The Demise of the New Parents' Old Self Image

Distorted by pregnancy, many mothers long for and work toward their pre-pregnancy body. Exercise and dieting in moderation are fine. But some people don't realize that dieting while nursing is not always easy. Further, the loss of too much extra body fat can weaken the flow and nutritional value of breast milk.

Although not common, some even opt for an early C-section (the Hollywood delivery) to avoid the disfigurement of a full-term pregnancy followed by vaginal delivery with its associated dreaded discomfort, pain, loss of control, and presumed indignity.

Most new mothers feel revealed and exposed; personal privacy is lost in a delivery. All modesty disappears with the audience present.

Many mothers do not feel very sexy after delivery. Gone is the self-image of an attractive, single woman with few responsibilities. Now, pushed out of shape, she is consumed with responsibility for an infant who is now totally dependent on his parents.

Fathers face a new reality as well. For several anxious reasons, they may gain weight during pregnancy; and the time to work it off is often unavailable after the baby arrives. Fathers are confronted with many new, inescapable responsibilities. Gone are the days of the single life, or even the life with just his wife.

The Father's Fragile Strength

Fathers, just like mothers, like to feel successful. They feel proud to have a nice family of their own. They feel protective and possessive. However, a new infant in the house can paradoxically be a challenge to those feelings. Increased responsibilities and demands for time are keenly felt.

For example, a father may feel burdened with financial concerns now that he may, even temporarily, be the sole breadwinner of the family. He may feel that he can no longer afford to take real risks in his career. He may have far less time and energy to pursue his career, and the fear of less success may worry him. *"Before, if anything happened it was just me and my wife, and she could survive without me. But now someone else is totally dependent upon my own success or failure."*

Crowded into his tightly managed life is the need to help his wife and child. Some fathers may resent the new demands posed by both wife and child; and some may find it hard to manage and empathize with the mother as she goes through hormone withdrawal during the postpartum period. A father may feel helpless when all attempts to calm her are unsuccessful. Anger, depression, and guilty feelings may follow. He wonders, *"What did I get myself into?"*

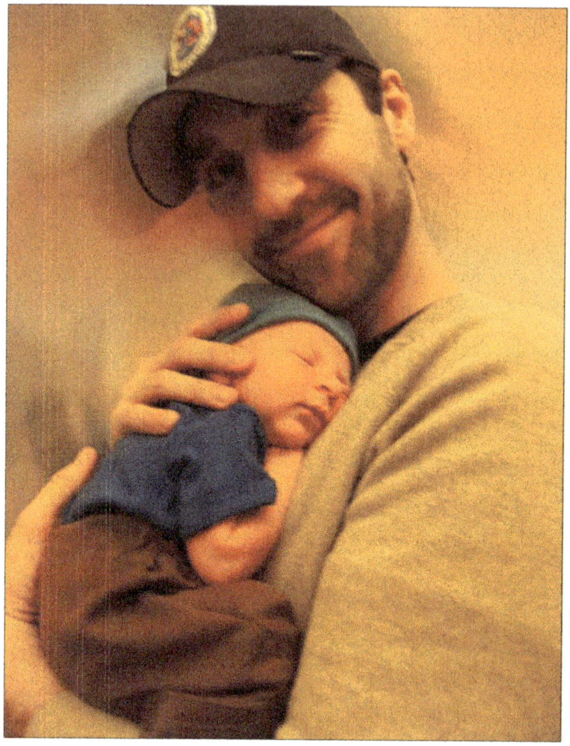

"It's nice. . .really nice."

Love and Hate

Sometimes even hate, while quite a strong word/feeling, toward the child erupts into conscious thought and confronts our love. Just as joy is mixed with sadness, a strange often-unacceptable mixture of love and hate occurs.

Parents feel the drive and desire for intimacy, closeness, love, and attachment with their new child. This force is expressed in the rapturous attempt for eye contact and recognition through sensual interactions involving vision, hearing, and snugly, soft secure embraces. Parents marvel as body features become more apparent and recognizable as coming from one parent or the other. Indeed, attachment deepens as we see ourselves in our children.

We then have the compelling instinct to see them happy. This ambition soon conflicts with the frustration that accompanies the child's development. The irritability of the high-strung temperament, difficult or unpleasant breast-feeding, or maddening colic all may cause anger and conflict with our love.

Hate for Love

A mother, father, and their six-week-old infant entered the office for a routine check-up. The mother kindly and quickly sought help, "I hope you don't mind but I have a lot of questions." Her many expressed concerns distilled into two essential worries: (1) their infant was not sleeping more than nine hours per twenty-four hours, (2) her nipples were becoming extremely sore, for when he was awake he screamed to nurse often. What was supposed to be sublime, blissful, warm, and pleasurable had become extremely unpleasant, painful... and deeply resented.

The mother, with discussion, realized that her concern over the lack of sleep of her child was connected to her concern for her own lack of sleep. Since her infant was staying awake, she herself was unable to sleep; she felt obligated to be with him during those "quiet, alert" times to seek his recognition. She repeatedly asked, "When will he smile at me, when will he recognize me?" She expressed an interest in discontinuing breast-feeding or, at least, in giving formula half of the time.

We discussed the pros and cons of this approach. She, teary-eyed and upset, blurted out that she was not enjoying being a new mother, that maybe she was not meant to be a mother, and that she had at times some very hateful feelings for this seemingly ungrateful and demanding infant. While sometimes cuddly and consolable her infant exhibited the characteristics of the "high-strung" infant (see Book I for more information about infant temperaments). (Also see the anecdote "Family Expectations, Part III")

One father reported shock when he suddenly fathomed the meaning of the words of a familiar lullaby he was singing while rocking and trying to console his slightly sick child. He was doubly shocked realizing the lyrics reflected his own peeved feelings at this infant who was rejecting all his best consoling efforts.

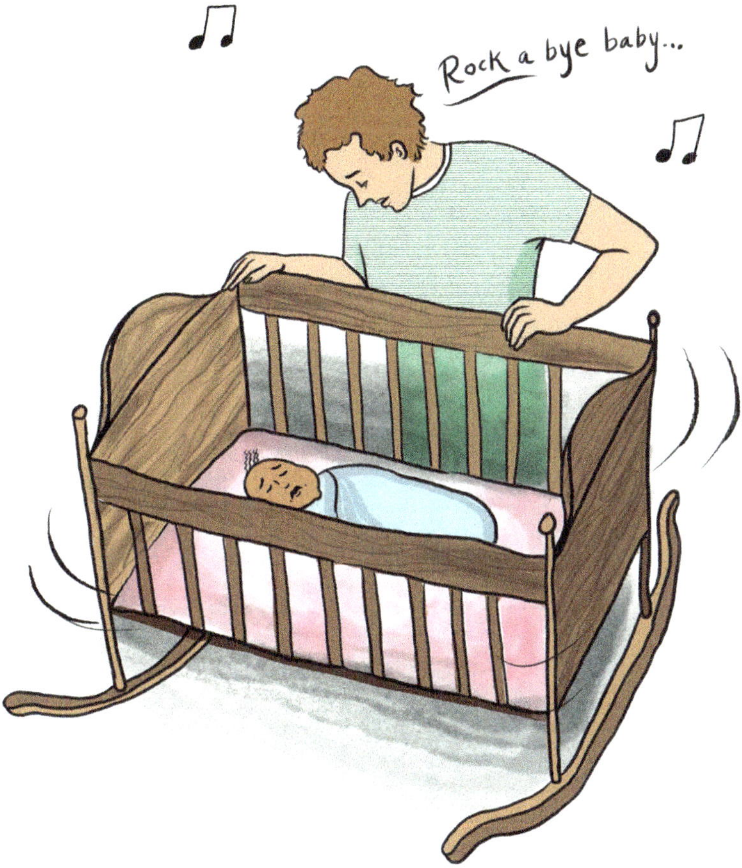

The lullaby:

"Rock a bye baby, on the tree top.
When the wind blows, the cradle will rock.
When the bough breaks, the cradle will fall,
And down will come baby, cradle and all!"

The Intruder Complex

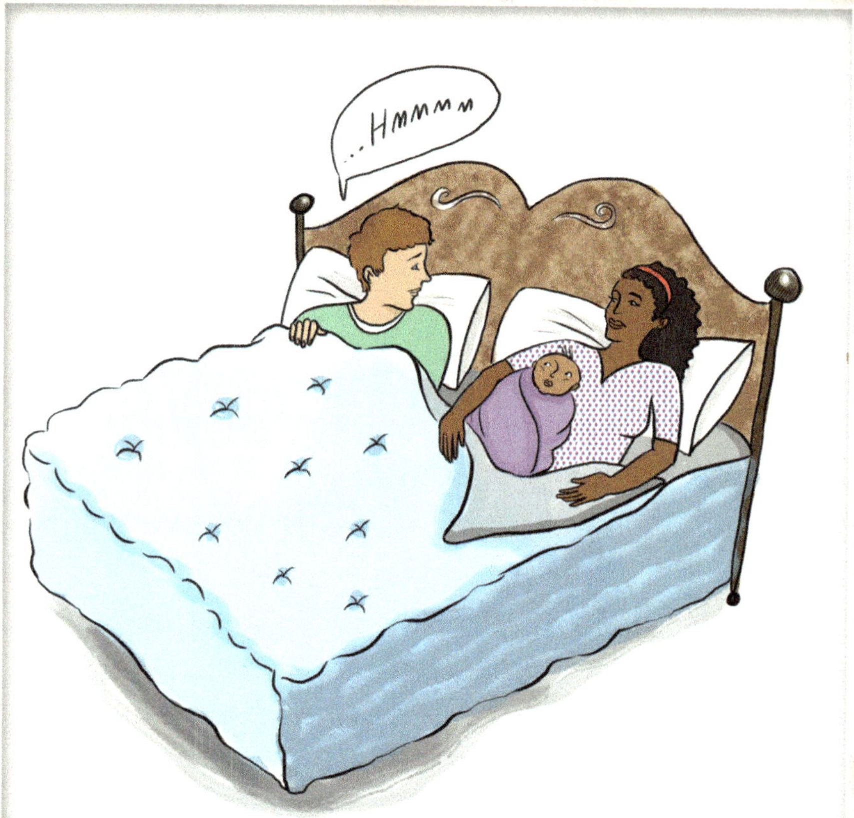

Chapter II:
The Intruder Complex BLOOMS

The Development of Intimacy

It's Not Automatic

While there is a drive toward intimacy, its actual development involves a dance that is not just automatically there for the taking. It is first cultivated through close conversation, whether that is talking about work, vacation, or what to eat for dinner. Over time, couples share more personal intimacies, including talking more about themselves and their families, sharing their vulnerabilities, and becoming physically intimate. They get to know one another and are more trusting of each other.

Eventually, a couple's love for each other outweighs the dread of being tied down, forsaking both youthful freedom and some of the bonds to their own parents. Then the couple's own family forms as romance is balanced with the wish for offspring, whether immediately after marriage or at some time in the future.

The Intimacy Vacuum

When you decide to try to become pregnant, or adopt, you are forced to face decisions and engage in preparations for something predictable but obscured by fog. The focus shifts away from you as a romantic couple.

Before this point, you had discussed the workplace politics, your next vacation, friends, and relatives. As a couple, you spent countless hours talking about books and films, inside jokes, favorite brunch places, and workout routines. Now, even if you do go out together, you are no longer discussing yourselves, what you are going to do, and your relationships with others. You are no longer the focus of your own conversations.

Instead, it's all about the baby-to-be: Where're you going to put this kid? Is the apartment large enough? Who will be the obstetrician? The pediatrician? What kind of furniture do you need? What car seat should you buy? And that is just the beginning of the list. While excitement abounds for this looming arrival, your life of intimacy is now on the wane.

The Unexpressed Growing Intrusion

The Slightly Tarnished Luster

Delivery is truly amazing and wondrous. New parents are thrilled and elated to the point of not even noticing they are missing sleep.

But exhaustion sets in after a few days. Visitors drop by. Well-wishers call in. Household chores become more apparent. If there are older siblings, they demand in, insisting for their own time. Emotions become raw, parents become a bit edgy from lack of sleep, demands from all sides, and, of course, hormone withdrawal. The profoundness of the change sinks in and, ever so slightly, tarnishes the luster of the unbelievable miracle.

An amazingly powerful, most often unconscious, feeling envelops parents: This new and longed-for infant has subtly, perhaps unexpectedly, intruded into the parents' own life of intimacy with each other, and each parent's sense of self. And parents respond.

This is The Intruder Complex. And it can blindside you.

For the Father

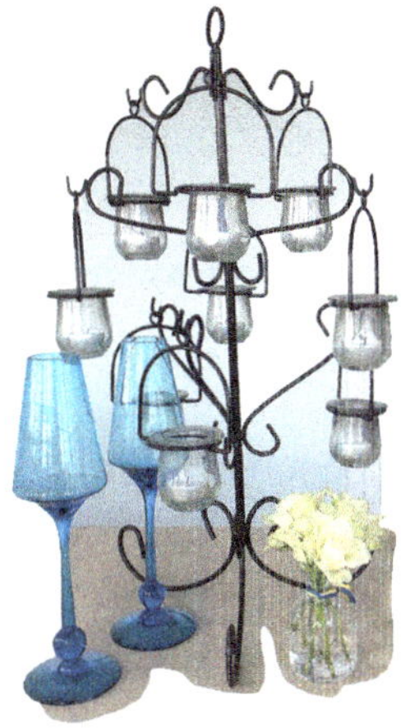

"Come on in. How was your day?"

Before the pregnancy, a couple might meet at home in the evening after work and spontaneously prepare dinner together, perhaps even with flowers, candles, music, or wine to their favorite serial TV show.

Erg! Abruptly a baby changes all that, and life quickly can settle into a series of continuous preoccupations.

Now a father may return home from his work to this not-so-uncommon scenario: He walks through the door and before his computer bag is set down, his wife pleads with him to care for the baby so she can get some needed sleep. He does what he can to help but may quickly begin to feel no one is showing any concern for him. As one father told me, *"Everyone is chattering incessantly about this infant, no one is interested in my needs. She used to hug me, kiss me, and invite, 'Come on in. How was your day?'"*

The father consciously or unconsciously often doubts, or at least wonders, if his wife/partner can continue to love him as much as she did before the baby arrived. And he can't complain; she has it worse!

How fathers manage these stressful situations and feelings depends on what their own parents modeled for them when they were infants and children and, also, on the support available from extended family.

Some researchers have categorized fathers into three groups: romantic fathers, who behave casually toward the child; career-oriented fathers, who feel burdened by the newborn; and family-oriented fathers, who develop an easy acceptance for their infants.

Clearly, family-oriented fathers who have felt, and successfully managed, the jealous feelings of having siblings may have more confidence and experience when confronting the feelings of exclusion and jealousy engendered by the Intruder Complex. In my observation, they come, more often than not, from emotionally healthy families of their own. Their fathers were good enough role models and both parents were emotionally there for them, offering security in good enough ways as they grew up. Family-oriented fathers typically enjoyed a good deal of time with their spouse before the baby arrived. (This bonding time helps a couple sustain its own bond of intimacy despite the intrusion of a baby)

However conversely, one or both parents of these family-oriented fathers may have been, or may have been perceived as having been, for one reason or another, emotionally unavailable. Then these new fathers may respond with the need and desire to become "family-oriented." As they talk in their minds to their new child they may find themselves saying, *"I don't want you to ever feel like I felt."* They then develop, or have created a mental/emotional vision, of what they want to be as an ideal father; and they then act toward that.

In my experience, career-oriented fathers aren't just burdened by work but may actually use their careers to avoid the overwhelming feelings that accompany fatherhood. *"She's not paying any attention to me, so why shouldn't I go to work where I can accomplish something, where I can be appreciated?"* These fathers often, while feeling pushed out as their wives take over, may be or become self-absorbed and want to attract attention, perhaps to get the attention that was lacking in their youth. So, they may seek attention elsewhere. (See *The Premature Invasion*, below.)

Indeed, a career-oriented father may have waffled between wanting and not wanting to have children in the first place. Or he may experience conflicting feelings between his desire to perpetuate his own genes (have a child) and the competition for the attention a new child requires.

The romantic father also feels the intrusion into his life of intimacy with his wife. The parents of these fathers often were not there for them as they grew up (whether emotionally or physically), leading them to expect more from their spouses than is realistic. In a sense, they are seeking from a spouse the warmth and feelings that were never or rarely received from their own mothers. In this scenario, the father's child may become a competing sibling, allowing The Intruder Complex to severely affect the relationships of the father with his wife/spouse and child.

Today many fathers seek an egalitarian presence in parenting. They want to contribute and be equally involved in the child care. But studies show that unless a problem exists, like prematurity, mothers tend to know more and subtly take over. The father can slowly begin feeling unneeded or not as important as he wanted to be.

Planned conception may be another complicating feature, one not easily forgotten by the father. While the father looks for romance and spontaneity, his wife may feel driven by a biological urgency to have a child sooner rather than later. In that scenario, the father may feel used like a "stud bull" and can come to resent scheduled sex. The romance is gone; sex is now mechanical. The desire, the wish, the thought of the longed-for child may now intrude into the couple's life of intimacy, even before conception. (See *The Premature Invasion*, below.)

The process of *in vitro* fertilization can be rewarding if it works immediately on the first try. But if repeated attempts are required, demoralizing frustration can become quite depressing. Each parent may unconsciously feel inadequate and if there is nowhere to talk about all of these feelings, sometimes they unfortunately might take them out on each other.

For the Mother

Mothers often express, *"Everyone wants a part of me. I hardly have time to be with my husband. The house is a mess and the relatives are coming. I'm exhausted. I'm not sure the baby is gaining weight. I don't feel like I'm doing well by anybody, especially myself!"*

Wishing to perform perfectly, yet devoid of energy because of new obligations, a mother may quickly become exhausted by routine tasks. She may be upset that she can't do what she had been capable of handling before. The house is disorganized and cluttered. Her husband wants her attention and so does her infant. She may have the overwhelming feeling of having to be available to everyone else and not having any time to herself. Her husband may need attention. But she feels that he, out of everyone around her, should be able to get along without her. And shouldn't he be helping her after all? *"He's a grown up. He's one of the parents, too. Right?"* She may even resent his attempts for attention feeling they get in the way of bonding with her new infant.

The baby requires her physically and emotionally—he is vulnerable and needy. The infant may be colicky, have a challenging temperament, or simply demonstrate the usual frustrations that accompany normal development. At the very least, he is demanding of her time with his need for love and constant nurturing.

And if her baby isn't perfectly content, the mother may become frustrated or angry since she has tried her best to make this infant happy. She may feel inadequate: the rejection of all her best efforts evokes worry, often followed by anger and resentment. The angry feelings toward this innocent infant can become frightening and disturbing for her. This is someone she thought she would love without conflict! In her mind, she must be a failure. *"I feel like I am being constantly evaluated...not only by others but also by myself."*

Pregnant women often fear that they will not love their baby. If the above scenario plays out, a mother might then worry that this fear is becoming a reality, leading her to feel guilty for not accomplishing her role perfectly. A self-fulfilling prophecy... perhaps one she created.

A mother's sense of fulfillment is just beginning. It is fragile. It can be easily undermined by a critical grandparent or by an annoyed husband who may be vacillating between asking for attention and distancing himself. A jealous friend or relative may be derogatorily judgmental, unsupportive, or may even refuse to visit. Thus, muffled anger and guilt are swirled into ecstatic love, all feelings stoking this murky vortex.

Paradise Lost

Another critical part of the parents' life of intimacy together is sex. At the beginning of pregnancy sex may be little changed, but eventually morning sickness and premature contractions might make it prohibitive. Delivery, while mutually thrilling, nevertheless necessitates a period of sexual abstinence. Even after the six-week "all clear" sign from the obstetrician, both parents are often tired, sleep-deprived, and preoccupied with worries and awe. Some new mothers are confronted, on top of everything else, with little to no sex drive.

A very long time, often actually years, may go by before the parents' sex life fully returns to its pre-pregnancy tempo. One mother shared her and her husband's experiences and feelings.

> ***"Finally!"***
> *I had a tear during my vaginal delivery. Let me tell you what a tear makes intercourse feel like, despite lubricants and very gentle lovemaking: Awful!!! Even going back for a visit to the obstetrician at six weeks postpartum to hear I was 'healed' from the episiotomy did not alter the fact that intercourse was painful.*
>
> *You can imagine how further left out my husband felt with my reluctance to resume sexual intimacy. We asked ourselves, is it ever going to feel right again?*
>
> *Coping with this probably enhanced our intimacy in the long run but it was very upsetting at the time. Curiously, and quite thankfully, it did not occur after our second son's birth.*
>
> *p.s. My husband and I text [message] each other. After our first night of enjoyable love, he wrote a simple text: "It Works!" He was patient and I appreciated it.*

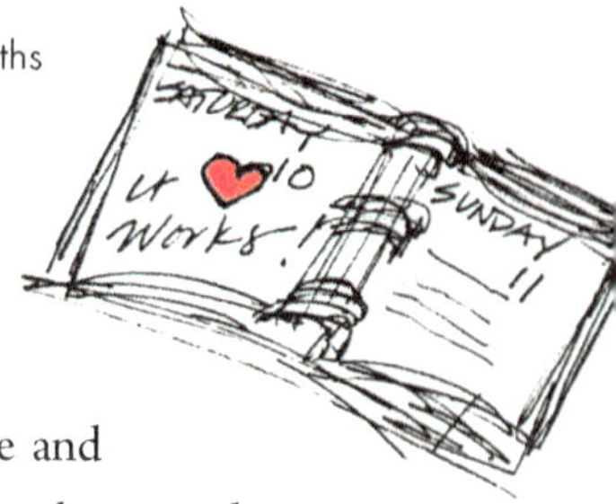

The Feeling Is Felt.

Out of all of this evolves a real sense that this longed-for infant has truly intruded into the parents' life of intimacy. Both parents feel less romance and concern for each other. The major dominating focus has become the new infant; he is front and center stage.

That is the Intruder Complex. It is not just a feeling; it is a reality. The new baby has intruded into his/her parents' lives and taken them hostage.

Intruder Complex Corollaries

For Mom

A mother may become jealous of the father. A father can sometimes, definitely not always, calm an infant more quickly than the mother, especially in the early months. Some mothers, feeling their infant's unhappiness, may become as upset as the infant and consequently be unable to reassure the child. Some mothers may be more anxious than the father. A breast-feeding infant may also associate the mother with nourishment so that when he's near his mother he roots and cries for the breast until calmed and satisfied. In his father's arms, he knows that breast-feeding is not possible and can then be more successfully calmed by other methods. (Remember *"Trying to Please Everyone, but Not Harry"* above.)

For Dad: Odd Man Out

Feeling proud but burdened with new responsibilities goes with the territory of fatherhood. A father now has less support from his wife. Despite being outwardly supportive about his wife's breast-feeding, he may consciously or unconsciously resent it. His infant now has his wife. The father's own possessive instincts may be challenged. His wife is now calling the shots. The father starts to feel like the "odd man out." Feeling unconsciously jealous, he can devolve from disinterested to detached and unloving toward his infant. In extreme cases, he may even have hostile fantasies toward his infant.

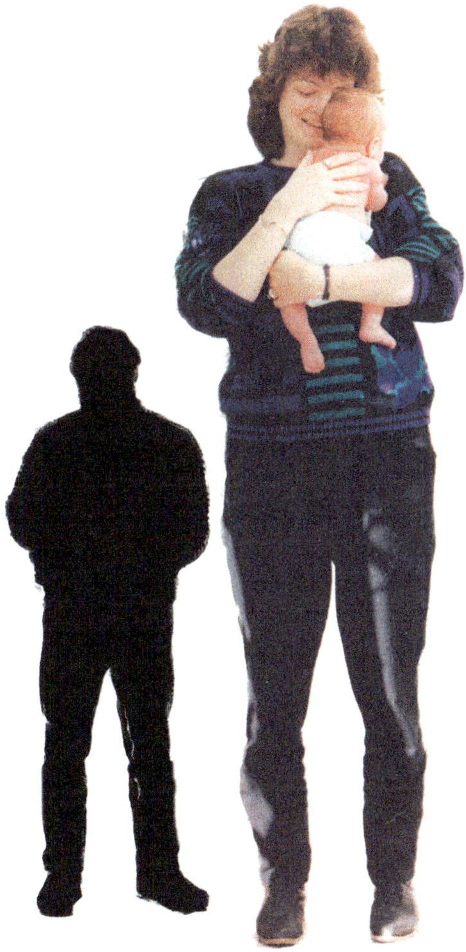

"Odd Man Out"

This episodic feeling, sometimes expressed but more often resentfully smothered, of "odd man out" is almost universal in varying degrees among new fathers. Yet a father may yearn for togetherness with his partner in this new, shared task. And the good news is this: If the couple can work through the infant's challenge to their intimacy, they can end up feeling even more emotional closeness than before. First, though, a father needs to get beyond feeling hurt and excluded, for only then will his involvement become more supportive of his wife and child and more gratifying for himself.

The Vacation-Reclamation Syndrome

When confronted with The Intruder Complex, a father is often determined to reestablish his relationship with his wife. He may sometimes choose a vacation to disrupt his wife's close, symbiotic (see glossary) attachment to their infant. I refer to this phenomenon as the "Vacation-Reclamation Syndrome." This is most common toward the end of the first year of the infant's life; however, occasionally a father may use an early vacation to dramatically and abruptly reclaim his wife's intimacy. The following story illustrates an extreme variation of this syndrome.

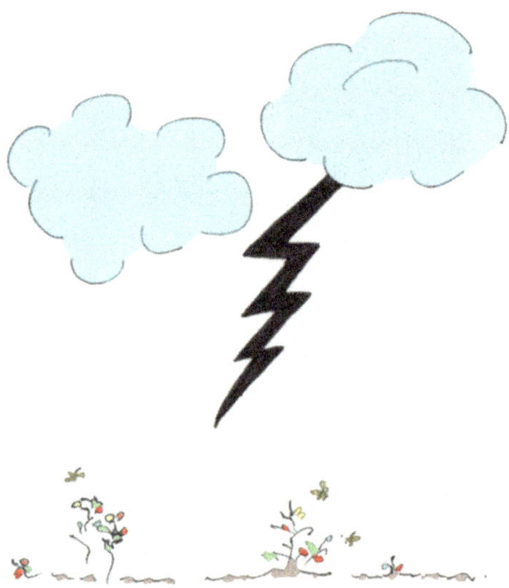

The Vacation... At Six Weeks?

Mr. and Mrs. Wyatt were both twenty-eight-years old when they had their first son, David. He was a delightfully warm, endearing little baby boy. To his mother's deep gratification, he breast-fed with ease. The initial few weeks were wonderful, not at all like the burden that many parents describe.

Suddenly, six weeks after baby David was born, like a thunderclap out of clear skies, Mr. Wyatt announced to his wife that he intended to take her, ***alone****, to San Francisco for a vacation in a few weeks. She was flabbergasted! Although stunned to almost complete silence, she managed to eke out of her mouth a refusal to go without bringing David along. Leaving her son behind would demand an abrupt weaning from the breast. Mr. Wyatt adamantly insisted that the trip was just for the two of them and, if she refused to join him, he was going regardless. He proceeded to arrange all the details. Expecting her to say no, he instead opted to invite an old college friend.*

Mrs. Wyatt felt terribly torn between her new son and her husband. After three days of true agonizing, she reluctantly informed her husband that she would accompany him on the trip. She had arranged to leave David with her parents and rapidly weaned him.

To her utter astonishment, the college friend accompanied them to San Francisco; Mr. Wyatt felt it would be impolite to un-invite him.

For the first months, the office visits were routine. The parents discussed no problems and acted as if all were well. Only later, after the vacation, was this story revealed. We discussed The Intruder Complex, the bonding and attachment process, normal symbiosis, and the "Kamikaze Mode" (see glossary). We analyzed the feelings that resulted from this almost vengeful vacation and the wrenching weaning it necessitated. We eventually talked about the father's instinct to be the main possessor of his wife's love, and her, and how their son had intruded into that relationship and how he now wanted it back for himself... and that was what the vacation-reclamation was all about!

This story is offered as an example of a phenomenon that can and does occur. It raises many questions, most of which will be addressed later in this book and in Book III. For now, suffice it to say that reclaiming intimacy is essential but doing it so early and so harshly can be problematic.

Interesting fact:
Charles Lindbergh (made famous for The Spirit of St. Louis) forced his wife to wean and go on vacation with him, alone, at approximately one month of age after the birth of each of their six children.

Its Power

Affairs

The Intruder Complex, initiated with pregnancy, is often a source of powerful conflicts between parents. Some conflicts are serious enough to lead to affairs, separations, and divorces in couples who had otherwise been, or at least appeared to be, quite happy prior to the pregnancy.

This is an often not-to-be-talked-about, thankfully infrequent, but occasional reality. The emergence of The Intruder Complex and the feeling of being "odd man out" can lead the father to seek sexual solace and illusory warmth and friendship elsewhere. Or a wife, feeling left alone or unattractive to her seemingly rejecting husband or to reassure herself that she has not lost her youthful ability to attract, may seek flattering compliments including a then reassuring sexual relationship...uncommonly, but sometimes, even with her husband's best friend.

While the following anecdotes are pulled together from multiple stories, they are not fiction. And it must also be said that, while The Intruder Complex operates here, The Intruder Complex is not an excuse for the following actions or behaviors. Rather, the two anecdotes are illuminated with the hope of preventive medicine and anticipatory guidance.

"Interesting fact" addendum:
The same Charles Lindbergh mentioned above also had three secret and separate mistresses in Europe and he sired seven children out of wedlock by them. This was unbeknownst to all those involved and only discovered after his death. (He would be in big trouble today given the Internet, iPhone tracking and videos, and social networking. Right? Perhaps not.)

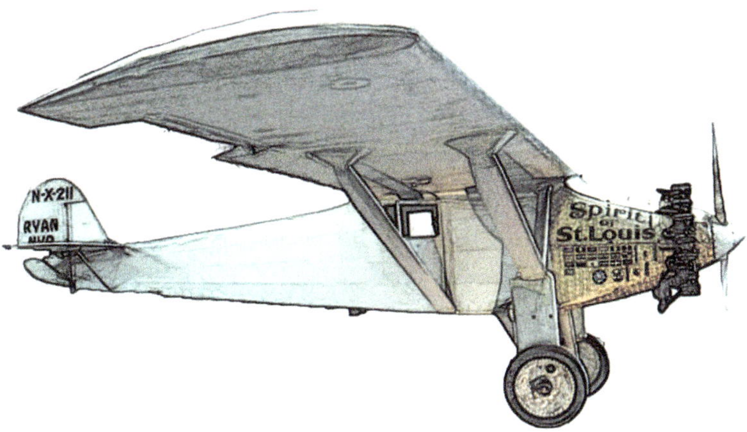

The Anniversary Bar
A mother came in for a checkup of her eight-month-old baby boy and shared the following story:

She had become suspicious that her husband was seeing another woman. One night, when he was late coming home on their wedding anniversary, she took her baby to see if her husband was at the local pub. Indeed, he was, and with another woman.

He came home with his wife and admitted to having had an affair with the woman. He claimed his good friend, who was also married and also quite macho, had challenged him to do it: "Come on out. You're acting like an old married man. What you need is an outlet."

Feeling remorse, he promised that it would never happen again and that he wanted very much for the marriage to continue. The mother wanted the marriage to work out but she didn't know how to get past her angry feelings toward him. She felt she now had two children.

The father felt abandoned, ignored, and insecure. He felt no one was paying attention to him anymore. He sought warmth and attention outside of his marriage and his new family. In addition, he felt a strong reluctance to give up the freedom of his youth. He explained that his own mother was not always there for him as he grew up and realized that he was looking for more from his wife than just a wife and a mother for his children; he was also looking for the nurturing that he lacked growing up. He felt insecure and anxious as a threatened father, almost and much like a competing sibling to his new infant.

The Premature Invasion

They both had large, extended families. They had gone together for two years and had been happily married for six months. He loved his wife, a lot. Being thirty-seven years old, she wanted to become pregnant as soon as possible. He was thirty-five. They discussed her wishes. He was reluctant to have children so soon after being married but acquiesced to his wife's wishes because he loved her.

For a number of months, they had perfunctory sex around the time of her ovulation; he complained but passively performed with her on top. He felt used, as if he were simply a "sperm bank." The spontaneity of romance was gone.

She concurred that sex-by-the-clock was tedious but she explicitly acknowledged feeling anxious that her biological clock was running out. She outwardly expressed she felt peer pressure. All her friends were having kids and were asking when was she going to have one. Feeling pressure to become pregnant, she pressed her husband into that passion. She lamented that it was difficult to get the idea of needing a child out of her head. It was there, forever driving her.

Eventually, the arduous sex resulted in pregnancy. Premature contractions then prevented sex. Increasingly the father felt excluded, left out. He didn't blame his wife; he just felt alone.

He had felt alone before. His own parents were aloof. His father had been highly critical and demeaning and his mother largely ignored him to pursue her career.

His work required travel. A younger, female colleague, who truly admired him, had to travel with him. It took only a few business trips together before they started an affair.

The child was born prematurely, which resulted in worry and the need for preoccupying attention. He also developed significant gastroesophageal regurgitation (GER) with pain and failure to gain weight. All of that preoccupied everyone: mother, father, and relatives.

The father felt more alone than ever. The mother and her relatives did not involve the father in the multiple concerns for their premature baby with significant GER. He had his work with its required travel. They tried to spare him from worry. The result, he felt unneeded. His life of intimacy with his wife was gone; all conversations revolved around this infant. Even their previously backbreaking sex life was now nonexistent.

He felt as though she were having her own affair: At first she was consumed with fertility, and now she was consumed with their new baby, who had serious medical problems.

His affair with his colleague flourished. They booked a long weekend together; he told his wife he was on a business trip. But, as they say, "fate intervened." The premature infant developed a major viral infection of his lungs in addition to complications from his GER, all of which halted his breathing. The mother called 911 and the baby was admitted to the Pediatric Intensive Care Unit of the local hospital. In trying to reach her husband, his wife learned there was no required business trip. Upon return he sadly and reluctantly confessed his affair.

She was wounded, and furious. She wanted to hurt him and immediately hired a divorce lawyer. He hung his head...said little.

A few days later, they came into the office with their infant and quickly related the above story.

The office transformed into a safe place where they began to sort out what happened. We discussed The Intruder Complex and the father's childhood experience of feeling emotionally alone. We discussed the mother's biological imperative and how this near obsession had been impossible to ignore. Each began for the first time to catch a glimmer of what the other had been feeling. The wife saw her husband's loneliness. The husband saw how his wife had been left to handle their infant's problems all alone. They realized they both had been feeling hurt and abandoned by the other. They saw how they both were angry and wanted to hurt the other.

With time and continued open communication, they became more thoughtful of each other; in fact, they became more considerate. They now complain that they argue much more but they acknowledge that arguing is better than the previous sullen, withholding silence. They are still married and even seem closer than ever.

Divorce, or "Uncoupling"

The above stories bring us back to one of the purposes of this book and its series: preventative psychiatry, as part of pediatric interventions. Many children (said to be as many as 60 percent) are, at some point in their lives, growing up in single-parent homes. Sometimes this is perhaps the only (or the best or, at least, the least destructive) outcome depending on the situation. Sometimes some vulnerable parents cannot weather the storm of The Intruder Complex; sometimes there are other stresses; sometimes coupling is chosen for the wrong reasons. So, sometimes uncoupling happens.

Perhaps parents can grow along with their children. Would that not be the better for everybody?

Would that not be the best for the child, if all in the family grew more, perhaps together and less apart, or at the very least grew somewhat from these experiences? Once you are a parent, there is no going back, not even with uncoupling. But if we can grow, perhaps even the disruption of uncoupling might be more caring and less traumatic on our children.

The Intruder Complex and other stressors can initiate divorce; but are in themselves not the cause of divorce. Stressors for marriage can also bring a couple closer as the couple masters them. If one wants to look for causes of divorce, you need to look at why people marry. More on that at another time.

However, the Intruder Complex can, if it remains in the unconscious, be unknowingly destructive. It is this author's experience that it is present, more or less, in every couple. Simply becoming aware of it, and the havoc it can wreak at times, brings it out of the unconscious and into the conscious; and that alone can help parents gain control of it thus allowing them to become better partners and parents. More on coping with The Intruder Complex will be presented in Chapter XI.

Its Longevity

I am not sure if the conflicts and the feelings of The Intruder Complex ever leave us. The following personal story illustrates the longevity of the Intruder Complex.

> ***Re-entry***
>
> *I went to a professional meeting in New York City with my wife, who works in a related field. We arranged for someone to care for our children while we were away. We had four wonderful days together, attending sessions during the day and spending evenings on the town. We ate well, went to plays, and had long talks, all of which reminded us of the time when we were students together enjoying our pre-child, romantic life.*
>
> *As the trip was coming to an end, I became depressed. We talked about it. I felt angry, then guilty and depressed that we had to return to our normal lives back home. Gone were the romantic four days and nights my wife and I had together. Gone was the hotel room we had to ourselves. I was depressed that life was not going to be as it had been during the time we were without children in New York.*

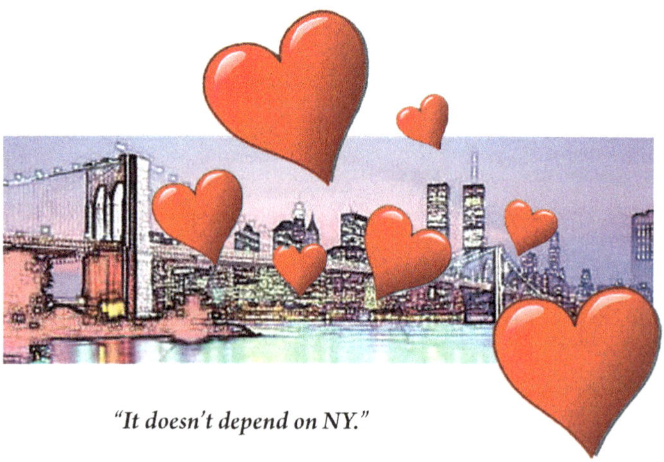

"It doesn't depend on NY."

> *I knew I was morose but I wasn't clear on why until we talked, and our close sharing opened the feeling of the loss of the intimacy we had shared in New York. I felt better after sharing my sadness because the sharing of it and the talking together helped me feel less alone. I could feel our intimacy again. And it was the kind of intimacy that didn't depend on being in New York.*

An old joke about a priest, a minister, and a rabbi arguing over when life begins highlights the endurance of The Intruder Complex: The priest was adamant that life begins at the moment of conception. The minister claimed, sometimes vehemently, that life is initiated only when the fetus is capable of living outside the womb with a sense of consciousness of its surroundings. Without this consciousness there was no life, he insisted. Finally, after an extensive and hot debate, the rabbi interrupted them, *"You two just don't understand. You are both wrong. You see, life begins only after the children have left for college!"*

That is The Intruder Complex.

An Historical Perspective

In the context of the study of the family, the term "complex" and the term "intrusion" have been used before. However, in each of its prior usages who is doing the intruding, and into which relationship or complex an intrusion occurred, has been considered from a different angle.

In 1938, a well-known French psychoanalyst, Jacques Lacan, was the first to use these terms in his treatise on *Family Complexes in the Formation of the Individual.* He used the term "complex" initially to describe "the Family Complex," or the family psychological structure *in toto,* which he noted was dominated by cultural factors after observing that the form and activity of the "family" often differed from one culture to the next.

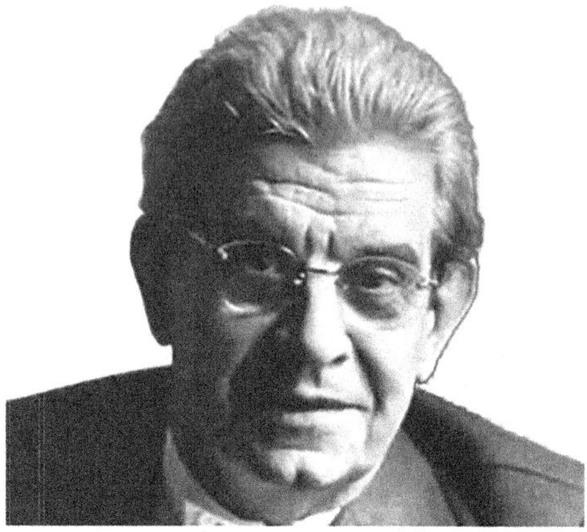

Jacques Lacan

The term "complex," however, then morphs in Lacan's almost metaphysical treatise on the family into the "complex" relationships that take place between two members within a family. He notes with astonishing clarity, "Complexes and imago have revolutionized psychology and, especially, the psychology of the family, which has shown itself to be the chosen terrain of the most stable and typical complexes." He then spends a lengthy time primarily on "The Weaning Complex" and "The Oedipal Complex."

The term "intrusion," also first used by Lacan, was limited in his treatise to the intrusion of a second sibling into the relationship between the first sibling and the mother, that is, Sibling Rivalry. Lacan used the term to refer to the first-born's feeling himself to be the "possessor" of the mother with the second-born child intruding into the first sibling's relationship with the mother. Lacan thus described the second sibling as the "usurper." He defines this as the "Complex of Intrusion," but limits this complex to sibling rivalry only.

However, any secure relationship existing within a family, especially the triad of today's modern Western family, can be strained by an intrusion. For example, a father may intrude into the relationship his wife has with their child and reclaim his intimacy with his wife by employing the "Vacation-Reclamation" Syndrome.

Further, any family can be disturbed by an intrusion from the outside. Grandparents, from the outside, can intrude into the family triad and parents' attempts to act as autonomous, independent caregivers. So, while Jacques Lacan discussed an "intrusion" as part of the Sibling Rivalry Complex, an intrusion can take place (and almost always does) in any relationship within a family with two individuals or more. And even if there are only two individuals, there can be an intrusion from the outside.

That being said, I can think of no better term than "The Intruder Complex" to label this major intrusion, that of the child into the intimate relationship between the two parents themselves.

How are

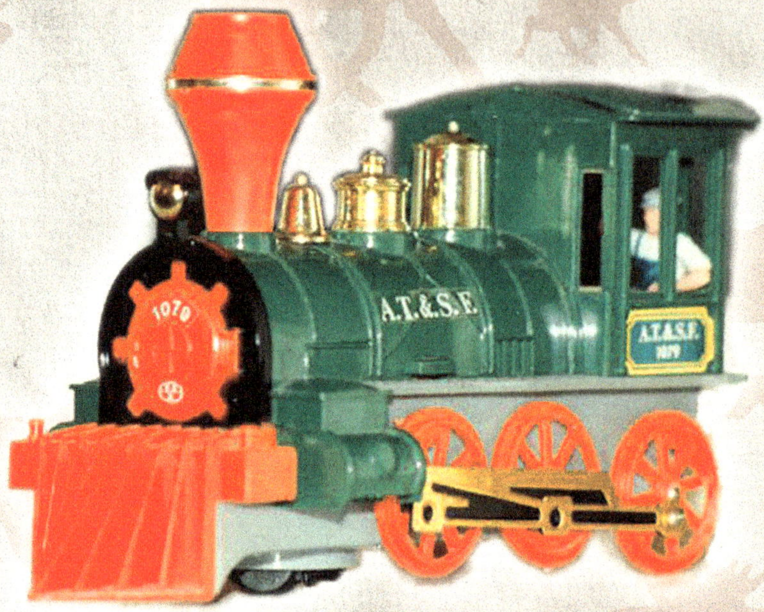

Breasts and Toy Trains alike?

Chapter III:
Breast Feelings

A Test of Confidence

Other complicated feelings can be part of this initial vortex just after a baby is born. Breast-feeding is clearly recommended for those who are able and where there is little risk. It can be a wonderful and natural experience. Breast-feeding may, on the other hand, present as an intrusion not only into a mother's sense of self but also into the parents' life of intimacy together. Also, the sense of one's own body and who "owns" it and how it looks or will look can influence the decisions of whether to breast-feed and for how long to breast-feed. While some mothers thrive with breast-feeding, others want their body back to themselves and feel losing their shape to the pregnancy was sufficient sacrifice. Also, for some mothers, sharing the breast with both husband and child can pose a conflict.

Tension/anxiety is a natural feeling when doing anything for the first time. During pregnancy, many expecting mothers are already concerned about successful breast-feeding. Some are so concerned that they don't even try. Others may feel confident in a supportive hospital setting but upon arriving home become more anxious. A mother expressed her worry: *"All of this depends on me. No one else can breast-feed this child. I don't know if I can do it. What if it doesn't work?"* This discomfiting feeling can actually interfere with breast-feeding.

How you were able as a child to master separation fears influences your sense of security (in this case with breast-feeding) as an adult. In other words, how secure, how comfortable are you when you are alone or doing something that no one else can do for you?

The happy and secure mastery of separation, the comfort with doing better than your parents, and how forgivingly versus punitively you strive for your own progress and not perfection are threads woven throughout this book and its series. These embedded fibers show their colors whenever you tackle something new or challenging as a parent.

The Grading System Returns

Book I in this series introduces the concepts of the Rite of Passage and the Grading System as they relate to pregnancy and delivery. We, and others, grade ourselves on how well we perform. Breast-feeding is no exception. The anxious question begins to form: *Can I be successful with this?*

One astute father asked me, *"Why is everyone so involved in just the process? Why aren't they focused on the result?"* The result, obviously, is to achieve the healthiest, happiest child possible, given the cards you are dealt, and to have a warm and wonderful attachment and experience with this child and, by doing so, enhance your happiness and relationship with your spouse. And you do that for both yourselves and your child. *"Love is other and self-regard."* But, it can be easy to lose sight of that when we get mired in "grading" ourselves.

Conflicts with Others

Others

Some approach breast-feeding with a religious seriousness, regardless of parents' feelings. They offer unsolicited advice and they blindly push for successful breast-feeding beyond any recognition of the mother's concerns or situation. This conflict often throws the new mother, who may be having problems with breast-feeding, into a quandary: she wants to perform well (the Grading System), and she feels incompetent when things aren't going well. The result? Guilt. This guilt can dampen her and her husband's experience of having a wonderful newborn. She may feel like she is failing in this rite of passage.

Everybody Is Entitled to My Opinion

"I have to tell you that women are the worst."

"My son is now 4 months old. I worked as hard as I could at breast-feeding. I went to my pediatrician and my lactation consultant. But my son had a neurologically dysfunctional suck. They, at our Children's Hospital, even x-ray videotaped to study my son's sucking and swallowing. He just could not latch onto the breast. So, I pumped. And then I gave him my pumped breast milk."

"I was at the lounge in Nordstrom's, giving my son pumped breast milk in a bottle. A woman suddenly appeared and said, 'You don't love your child! Why are you bottle-feeding him?' I collapsed in tears, truly devastated. This on top of everything I had tried and gone through. I asked myself, why do women do this to each other? It took me back to the sixth-grade mean girls' cliques."

The temperament of the infant and his brain's organization of his suck can cause problems, as can an engorged breast or an inverted nipple. Other, non-medical complications include the mother's sense of security and confidence, "breast feelings" as described in this section, the criticisms of others, the mother's employment situation, and the demands of the rest of the family.

Another story about "others" as blind and relentless zealots comes from a *Washington Post* article by Emily Wax-Thibodeaux (*"Why I don't breast-feed, if you must know,"* October 13, 2014, Health and Science section). The author required a double mastectomy with reconstruction for breast cancer at the age of thirty-two, followed by chemotherapy. Five years later she and her husband opted to get pregnant and they joyously delivered a wonderful baby boy. The hospital lactation consultants visited, *"You really should breast-feed."* They would not leave her alone. She was trying to enjoy her bliss; she was happy to be alive and have a healthy child. Her breast cancer surgeon said, *"No group should make a woman feel guilty about the decisions she made... or make her feel inadequate about not being able to lactate."*

And the Stories Go On

"A dear friend of mine adopted an infant at his birth. She was given a lot of criticism and side eye when people saw her feeding her newborn formula from a bottle. She should not have to explain to a stranger his adoption and her subsequent choice to formula-feed her baby."

Remember what's most important is not the process...it is the result. The goal is close, nurturing, warm relationships that are enjoyed by all. So sometimes breast-feeding is easy and wonderful but sometimes it is not, and sometimes it is not possible. Long ago there used to be an adage on a drift-wood plank above the entrance to a once popular 1960's delicatessen on Pennsylvania Avenue in Washington, DC:

As you wander through life
Remember your Goal
Keep your eye on the Donut
and not
the Hole

The Mother's Mother

Not uncommonly, a mother may feel inept and insecure compared to her own mother, whom she views as having been successful in the motherhood role. When a new mother attempts self-mastery, a fear of being equal to or even more successful than her own mother can feel like a betrayal or loss of her own mother. These powerful feelings can hinder successful breast-feeding. (See the anecdotes *"The Ultimate Loss Perceived"* and *"Hypnotic Suggestions and the Wildest of Dreams"*). More on this further on in this book.

The Husband

Fathers often feel excluded from the closeness inherent in a nursing relationship. They may also become unconsciously jealous, especially if the infant is a breast-fed boy.

"You can't be serious!"

I am serious. Just read this true story:

"Toy Trains"

One father, with a three-year-old boy, proudly announced to me that his wife was pregnant again, this time with twin boys.

Attempting to practice a little anticipatory guidance, I initiated a discussion of jealousy and The Intruder Complex since he would soon become the father of three boys, two of whom would soon be breast-feeding. (His wife had breast-fed their first child for two years; and she was going to breast-feed these twins as well.) About three minutes into my oratory, he interrupted me with a smile and proclaimed,

"Dr. Peebles, that reminds me of a joke."

"It does?" I responded, hoping for a professionally enigmatic expression on my face.

"How are breasts and toy trains alike?"

A quiet flush spread across my face and I admitted to being truly taken aback, "I don't know, how are they alike?"

"Well, they're both designed for kids and the fathers like to play with them!"

Wow! Well I guess the above jest poignantly represents many fathers' feelings. Part of a couple's love for each other is a sense of security in possessing the "undivided" love of the other person. However, when a new infant has the mother's breast while the father (often but not always) does not, and the parents' sex life is on the wane, very understandable but unconscious and unspoken jealousy can result. But humor, like the above joke, and the ability to share good-naturedly are wonderful adaptive responses useful for parental survival.

The Experts

The nurses, the doctors, the lactation consultants, lactating mothers, doulas, and the American Academy of Pediatrics all strongly recommend breast-feeding for the first six to twelve months of life, especially for premature infants. It is natural, it is cost-effective, and it is usually safe. However, it is not always easy, and rarely can be risky. All of us strongly recommend, encourage, and support breast-feeding but we should not judge, or castigate, those who do not, cannot, or opt not to breast-feed. And saying to all expectant mothers that *"breast-feeding is the most wonderful gift you can give your baby"* may not be supportive of or helpful for those mothers who cannot. In fact, life and love may be the most wonderful gifts you can give your baby. (See the anecdote, *"Everybody is Entitled to My Opinion,"* above.)

Studies that start with bias either from the formula companies or from breast-feeding advocates are not always easy to evaluate. The bottom line: In underdeveloped countries, formulas should be prohibited, as they are by United Nations' mandate. Also, premature babies have far fewer problems if receiving breast milk, even donor breast milk. Breast-feeding or breast milk is strongly recommended in that instance. However, in developed countries with refrigeration, improved formulas, and better management of the viruses that cause infant diarrhea, there are only slight and quite questionable differences between full-term breast-fed and formula-fed infants. There should be empathetic support, with no negative judgments, for those mothers who do not, cannot, or opt not to breast-feed for a host of more-often-than-not understandable reasons.

THE GIVING UP OF SELF

Drained

"I feel a wave of depression when he nurses. It is hard to share your body. I cried to my baby, 'You've had my body for nine months and now you want more!' I feel drained."

Many mothers love to breast-feed, some for an extended period. (See the anecdote *"Two Blue Barrettes,"* in Book IV. See also the cover and related article from *Time* magazine, May 21, 2012, for a great picture/study of this phenomenon.) But not all women do, and especially not indefinitely.

A mother may feel tied down, drained, and pushed out of shape. She may have lost her figure and self-image. As one mother graphically expressed it, *"I feel like an empty tit!"* A mother may believe dieting and weight loss are not allowed. She may feel she is sacrificing herself, yet again.

Often, after breast-feeding for a year or so, a mother will feel that she has sacrificed herself enough. She wants to wean and resents the infant's relentless tugs at her shirt. She yearns for her infant to calm himself and not suckle on her for each-and-every need for solace. These feelings are natural; they are part of "separation-individuation" conflicts (see glossary). They are understandable and should not be made worse by feeling guilty about them.

On the other hand, some mothers may be reluctant to wean. They may be unconsciously anxious about their own separation-individuation. (See the anecdote *"Two Blue Barrettes,"* in Book IV), and worry about resuming pre-baby intimacy with their husband and moving forward with their role as mother, wife, and person. This may especially be true if the mother perceives this to be her last child, as it may mean an end to an important phase in her life.

Weaning is a separation and individuation. It, for both parent and child, is a giving up of a phase of life and going on to another. There is joy and marvel in the accomplishment and growth, but a sadness in letting go and leaving that part of life behind.

In some cases of prolonged breast-feeding, a mother may yearn to remain the sole source of solace for her infant. While the ostensible goal is the infant's happiness, the infant, in fact, may then remain fearfully (as opposed to comfortably) attached to the mother. More on this in later books.

> ***The Drippy Mess***
> *"I don't like going to bed and making love with my husband with nursing pads and a great big cotton bra! I don't feel very sexy, and I feel I am really unattractive to him. I also don't like going to bed without the bra. If I do, I wake up all sticky and wet and messy. But I have not really discussed it with him. I don't know how he feels."*

Many nursing mothers don't think of themselves as sexually appealing to their partners, which may provide another reason to avoid sex. They have no idea how a partner might perceive the situation—the partner may, in fact, be experiencing a sense of sexual deprivation beyond any time frame they had anticipated. Ironically, they may be the one feeling rejected.

When a mother feels like a "drippy mess" (or any other understandable loss of her youthful sexual or personal attractiveness), it is thoughtful for the spouse to give loving compliments regarding her looks or dress. That's kind of nice. We often don't realize how much that is appreciated.

Sensual Feelings

This topic is sometimes difficult for most people to discuss. The hormones, particularly oxytocin, evoked by nipple stimulation and important to the milk ejection reflex (the "let-down reflex") are also involved in sexual orgasms and, studies show, in the touching required for bonding and attachment (see The Biochemistry of Love, and Bonding in Chapter VI). A nursing infant will thus stimulate in the mother not only milk secretion but also the hormones responsible for sexual feelings including the vaginal lubricating secretions. So, once the initial soreness is gone, many mothers can be sexually stimulated, at least to some extent, by a suckling infant.

While some may enjoy this, others feel guilty, thinking they may be perverted. These guilt feelings may restrict the milk ejection reflex and decrease breast milk flow. In others, it may lead to early weaning to avoid these feelings. To get those thoughts out of her brain a mother may then suddenly wish to reactivate sexual relations with her husband. Other nursing mothers, more commonly, may not desire or have sex with their husbands until their infant is weaned. During the nursing period, they may feel it is too difficult to be sensually intimate with more than one person at a time. Some mothers, anticipating this, opt for formula-feeding to avoid the conflict.

Thus, much like having the infant in the parents' bedroom (if not the bed itself), breast-feeding may severely cut into the parents' life of intimacy together, including their sex life. Not infrequently a mother may welcome breast-feeding to avoid other demands on her and her body from sexual intimacies with her spouse. Avoiding spousal intimacy results in one less intrusion into her joyous bonding with her child. Breast-feeding enhances closeness with the infant. However, for some mothers it is hard to share that intimate closeness with more than one person at a time.

Nipple Territory...and Breast Boundaries

Nipple Territory

> ***How Many People Can Be All Over Me?***
> *"I really miss the days before he was born. My wife and I were just buddies and would hang together. Now there is no time. But, recently we did have five days of vacation alone together, and that was great.* **(Note the Vacation-Reclamation Syndrome, above.)** *My sister kept Aaron, since he is now nine months old. I really grew up with cold parents, and now I love just hanging with my wife. We were talking the other night. Like many nights, I wanted to make love. But she was tired and also said that during the day our son was all over her. At night, she told me it was nothing personal but she didn't want me all over*

her. She wanted her body back to herself. She wanted a break. But she told me something else. She's breast-feeding, you know. Now that turns out to be a problem. During our lovemaking, she really doesn't like me to go for her breasts and especially her nipples. She feels that is little Aaron's territory now and not mine. She says it messes up her sexual fantasies. Now that's really hard for me but I can understand it. It was nice that we could talk openly, like the buddies we are. And it was nice to have that vacation time together alone. Little Aaron, when he first saw us come in the door after being away, was miffed for about forty-five seconds before he dove into our arms."

Breasts for the Father, Formula for the Kid

"I didn't breast-feed him. I wasn't comfortable doing that knowing that my husband was seriously concerned. I also was not comfortable with the idea of both my husband and my baby at my breasts. Formula was the solution. We were both very comfortable with that. So, I just put our child on formula."

Women who successfully breast-feed may encounter problems with sexual intimacy. During sex, a mother's usual sexual fantasies may be abruptly disrupted as she thinks of her suckling infant. It may be especially difficult to share the breasts with both husband and infant. Or she may feel, *"My husband can have my breast but the nipple belongs to the baby,"* since it may be upsetting to her to let her husband suck on it as he previously did. This common but unspoken feeling can persist for years, if not decades, beyond weaning. It incorporates much of what's been talked about already: guilt and confusion followed by intrusion into sexual fantasies and sexual enjoyment.

Once again, this is The Intruder Complex, which can lead to the partner feeling rejected and hurt. He may insist that his wife wean, or attempt to force weaning with the "Vacation-Reclamation Syndrome" described earlier (also see more on the Vacation-Reclamation Syndrome in Book III). To reclaim intimacy between mother and father is good for the child; it is an enhancement for an intact family. But a "vacation-reclamation" at six weeks is quite harsh. It is far better to wait for bonding and attachment to evolve and become established. So sometimes, a weekend alone may be the only way a mother and father can resume their former life of intimacy without the disrupting presence of their infant. And that can be done toward the end of the first year (give or take some months here or there).

Oral sex and Masturbation

One mother related her solution: She was happily breast-feeding when her baby was eight months old. She shared the feelings that the breasts and nipples belonged to her infant daughter. She kept her husband and herself happy...with oral sex.

Some mothers can resume sex of any kind right after delivery, even while breast-feeding. However, many experience these territorial feelings and have a hard time navigating the boundaries of what belongs to whom. We are raised to be monogamous; but now there is a threesome. Not always easy.

Both parents can feel abandoned and alone. The mother may feel that her needy infant consumes her. Her husband should be strong, he is not a needy infant, and he can survive for a while without her.

But can he? While she may know that he is sexually deprived and unhappy, she may not feel she has the energy to satisfy his needs. She may say to herself, *"But I do expect you to understand and to be faithful to our child and me. After all you are the grown-up, right?"*

The husband may be feeling odd-man-out. Everyone seems consumed with this new infant. His sex life is nonexistent, he has no one to talk to, and his wife doesn't even have time or energy to give him a simple hug. And so, he also forgets to give hugs. Or the possessive part of love may dominate his unconscious thinking: *"This is great but you are mine and we are going on a vacation and you need to wean."*

Well, it is sometimes hard for all of us to share, and realize that maybe it is not simply all about me. And if we have a hard time with that, it's worth looking at. It may be from our growing up with a perception of an unfulfilled need. And now we demand that it be fulfilled?

In some instances, a husband's solution may be to self-sooth with masturbation. But she may resent that, feeling jealous of his self-indulgence. This conflict, again, illustrates the complexities of The Intruder Complex.

When and if a marriage reaches this point, it is good for spouses to share and talk, out loud or maybe even in writing to each other. See Concepts for Coping.

Nursing Another's Infant?

"Wet nursing," not merely a common practice before formula existed, was in some instances a necessity. Before the 20th century with its formulas, a baby's life was at risk if a mother was unable to produce sufficient milk. So, a wet nurse was a salvation. The practice of wet nursing is ancient and multicultural: It is mentioned in the Bible; the Islamic prophet Muhammad was wet nursed; and it was quite common in ancient Rome.

It is an uncommon occurrence these days in our Western culture. But sometimes a new mother may require, for example, hospitalization. If her infant has been exclusively breast-fed, the infant may completely refuse a bottle. A friend who is also breast-feeding may offer to help out and breast-feed this mother's infant. Sometimes, two couples may go on a summer vacation to the beach together. Both mothers will be breast-feeding and wonder, *"Why don't I breast-feed both infants while you relax in the sun, and then you can do the same for me while I am on the beach."* Very low birth weight prematures may require donor breast milk to avoid severe life-threatening complications.

Many mothers would consider breast-feeding another's infant unconscionable, feeling understandably disturbed by the thought of sharing the close intimacy of breast-feeding with someone else's infant...perhaps a breakdown in boundaries, a taboo, or possibly unsanitary with a sharing of bodily fluids. Yet, sometimes it is practical or necessary to help another breast-feeding mother in distress. However, doing so may result in complex feelings arising from the shared intimacy of breast-feeding. Regarding sanitation: breast milk is safe unless there is active mastitis or the mother has a chronic active viral infection such as HIV or hepatitis B. But a mother with a risky chronic viral infection will know that from her pregnancy and delivery studies and, more likely, not be breast-feeding at all because of that.

Nursing an Adopted Infant or an Infant from a Surrogate Mother

The glue of bonding and attachment is touch: kissing, nuzzling, holding, and caressing are essential to bonding (see the Biochemistry of Love, and Bonding in Chapter VI). Breast-feeding is another form of intimate touch. So, while it is not necessary to breast-feed an adopted infant, it can be useful for enhancing bonding along with the other more common modalities of touch. It can sometimes induce lactation (usually not). But the closeness and the wonderful touch are felt as the suckling induces the hormones of bonding. It is also nice to take a bath with an adopted infant, thus feeling that warm, wet closeness and skin-to-skin caressing. This bath can be experienced with both parents.

Other

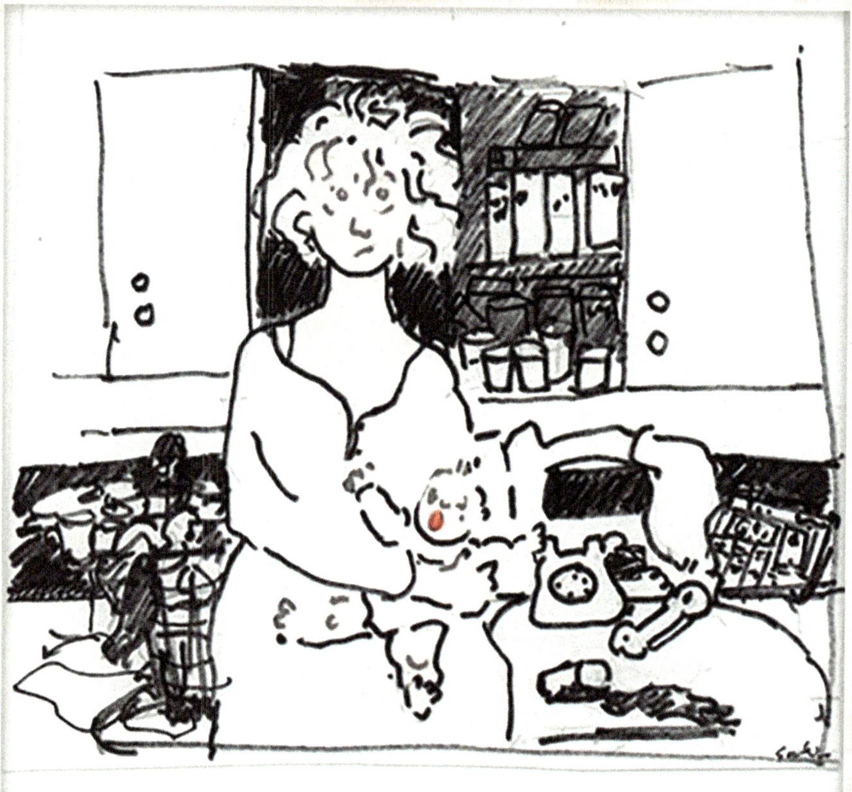

Gusts !

Chapter IV:
Other Gusts

Denial of Difficulties

***Family Expectations, Part III* (Continued from Book I)**
Mrs. Sin said, "I was very upset when we first came home because I thought all babies slept all day long without making a noise. I yearningly thought, 'now I can do all the recreational reading I want.' But our daughter doesn't sleep. She sleeps even less now."

Mr. Sin added, "Well, she sleeps at night, we had better be thankful at least for that!"

She continued, "She would cry all day and all night. I couldn't do a single thing. I was ready to give her back."

He commented, "That was a rough couple of weeks...very, very tough."

The Deterioration of Joyful Anticipation

This Was Supposed to Go Fine
"We weren't supposed to be concerned. All of this was supposed to go fine. I don't understand. I was looking forward to being only thrilled. Now we have jaundice. And I am not sure he's nursing well. And he's sleeping all of the time."

With any rite of passage, we hope, perhaps expect, that all should go well. But inevitably some little glitch might arise that can detract from the joy of anticipating that all will go well. But just because something did not go *perfectly*, or even *as expected*, does not mean that it did not go well. (See "Wish versus Reality" in the index.)

The Failure of Perfection

(See the anecdote "*Trying to Please Everyone, but Not Harry.*")

The world of adults, the world before pregnancy and delivery in which the mother was accustomed to feel in control, may seem gone. Now a mother may fall to pieces as she tries to do everything for everyone. She wants adult things for herself, a clean house and nice meals for her husband, all while having warm, loving, and nurturing feelings for her baby. Everything is give, give, give...and little time is left for her.

Failure to do everything perfectly can create guilt. The mother's self-given "grade" in this Rite of Passage of Parenting drops lower; and she worries that others see her failing, further eroding her self-confidence. She may blame herself, her husband...or even her baby! (See "*Family Expectations, Part III,*" above; see also Chapter X on Guilt, and Chapter XII on Blame, not to mention the Homunculus Phenomenon.) Her partner may not be as available as he was in the early weeks. She may become depressed with a foggy sense of loss. She may feel jealous, angry, and resentment at her partner's ability to escape. She believes and then resents that other new mothers may be going out, back into their old clothes, making love with their husbands, out playing tennis again, or returning to work with aplomb.

"Everyone says it's going to be fine and wonderful. They say, 'Isn't it wonderful you have a baby!' and 'Don't you look good! Take a little time and put on some makeup,'" cried one mother. She lamented the lack of at least a bit of the quiet sympathy she had wished for. A mother can find herself upset over sore nipples, leaky breasts, hair falling out, red eyes, body shape with sagging stretch marks, and her inability to get things organized. When the first dinner guests arrive, or the bris or christening occurs, things may not go perfectly. A mother may then fear appearing incompetent in front of her relatives and friends. All of this continues to be accentuated by utter exhaustion from the feelings, the work, and the lost sleep. One mother insightfully touched on it: *"When you're this tired, when 'your tank is empty,' you lack your usual resilience to deal with all of this stress. Any one or two of these feelings could be manageable if you are well rested, probably, but not when you are already* ***drained****."* This Rite of Passage may not be going as well as envisioned.

These challenges test a mother's self-confidence. Sometimes a mother, especially one who has been raised dependently, will become more dependent upon her husband. While unable to express his own worry that he may not be able to manage everything, the husband may become frightened, even crushed, by this additional burden on top of his own problems.

These parental inadequacy feelings emerge from multiple sources: giving up a part of one's self in taking on a new role, the worry of being alone but expected to handle all things, being raised dependent and not independent, and unconsciously fearing the "ultimate separation." (See "*The Ultimate Loss Perception*," below.)

Mothers who felt the "glow" and pride of pregnancy may be sad that the pregnancy is over. They can even become depressed, especially if the child has a temperament or gender other than what they had imagined and desired. Under these circumstances a mother may have dreams that the child is totally separated and lost from her.

The Loss of Control

About five to seven days after delivery, a mother may find herself uncontrollably weepy or easily upset with no apparent reason. This widely described sensation occurs simultaneously as the high levels of hormones required for maintenance of the pregnancy leave her body. It is, in effect, a drug withdrawal. One's best bet is not to fight it but to simply ride it out or, if severe to the extent that a mother can't function, seek help from the obstetrician. The weepiness is also regressive, which as described in Book I can commonly create fear. Sometimes a daily dose of vitamin B_6 along with a mild diuretic can be remarkably helpful. For others, an antidepressant and supportive psychotherapy may be essential. (Also see Chapter XI, Postpartum Depression)

Also, it is not always possible to have control of this new infant. He may be demanding, not easily scheduled, requiring one diaper change after another, or at times inconsolably colicky. For those who are used to being in control, all of this can be shockingly difficult, particularly if the parent has a temperament with low frustration tolerance, or is under a postpartum depression.

The Abandonment of Invincibility

Fears are forever. They come with love. The fears start with pregnancy and evolve after delivery. There are worries of Sudden Infant Death Syndrome, serious illness, bad teachers and baby sitters, or strangers offering candy on the neighborhood streets. Parents worry about older children getting into a car with a friend who has been drinking. Such fears continue to evolve constantly throughout our beloved children's lives.

Worry and the wish to control, as a way to avoid guilt, sadness, fear, and anger, are the inevitable consequences and burdens of parenting. When you love someone, you are doomed to worry. In other words, you are no longer invincible ... try as you may.

The Crisis of Change

Career Mother

Mrs. Olevan was thirty-six years old when she had her first child. Mothering came easily to her. She was warm, nurturing, and always available. However, when her baby was about one month old, she became extremely depressed, feeling alone. She suffered through this down period by herself, eventually fighting her way out of it with busywork, getting out with her new infant (with whom she was very much in love), and returning to her work part-time.

Mr. and Mrs. Olevan had initially put off having children because they married (relatively) late as both were focused on their careers. They were now financially more than quite solvent. They moved out of the city to a suburb to experience a grass lawn and a house with sufficient room for two children.

Mrs. Olevan had never thought that she could take to suburban life. She initially lacked interest in her neighbors, thinking that she had little in common with them. She soon discovered that some were not so bad; in fact, she shared many, but not all, of the perspectives of the other neighborhood mothers.

Another baby came along when her first child was almost two years old. With this second infant, she did not suffer the depression she had after her first child but instead enjoyed her situation very much.

With Mrs. Olevan, after her second child was a few months old, we looked back and discussed her depression after her first delivery. What was the difference, why was she not depressed after the second delivery?

Now that she had some distance from it, she could share her feelings. She thoroughly enjoyed her previous work. She loved her career and had cultivated friends within it over many years, most of whom did not have children. After she had a child, her friends continued on with their own careers while Mrs. Olevan was home with her new baby. When she met socially with her friends from work, the discussion focused on where the next vacation was to be, their latest partner(s), the current office gossip, et cetera. She was alone in the room with them and they were bored and unconcerned about the colic that was constantly on Mrs. Olevan's mind.

With the lack of any mutual interests, Mrs. Olevan and her friends slowly drifted apart. She felt a deep loss of the relationships she had cultivated for more than fifteen years. She was envious of their exciting, continued successes in their careers and depressed that she no longer could compete with them in her part-time status. Mrs. Olevan, suffering these losses of friends and self-image, eventually became significantly depressed.

That kind of sadness described above is increasingly common, as more women have enjoyed the opportunity to develop careers. An intensely perceived loss of previous roles, such as career woman, makes it difficult to adapt and accept decreased expectations and aspirations.

Taking on the new role of parent presents a big change to the mother who has a career. There is ambivalence around being a stay-at-home mother (even if temporary). The parent feels losses and gains. This simultaneous mixture of joy and sadness can be confusing and upsetting.

The Ultimate Loss Perception... and Success Neurosis

Another reality tale, one I would like to tell even though it at first glance may be perceived as unbelievable, perhaps even a tall tale, depicts the sadness and difficulties from the most fundamental loss perception that may transpire. This loss, since it is unfortunately most often felt unconsciously, is hard to control. Usually, it is simply experienced and realized late, and only with reflection after time has passed. It happens, to more-or-less extent, in all of us as we mature through this rite of passage. Having a child means we are the parents; and we are no longer the children. We have arrived into adulthood. But does this new non-dependence, this stand-on-our-own-two-feet-as-a-parent mean we have lost our own parents as parents?

The Ultimate Loss Perceived

Mrs. Appleton delivered a healthy, beautiful baby girl named Lisa. All was going quite well with breast-feeding until Lisa was three weeks old. She began to lose weight. All efforts to salvage breast-feeding were unsuccessful. Lisa was slowly switched to formula (with reluctance from her mother, physician, doula, and lactation consultant) in order to reestablish growth and assure mental development.

I was puzzled as to the cause of this particular early weaning, which was required to prevent Lisa's further failure to thrive. I (and all pediatricians) had, unfortunately, seen it previously in many other patients. We started to talk about it, but Mrs. Appleton preferred to write it down as a letter. The following is an exact copy of that letter (with names changed, and with permission).

"It was not possible for me to begin nursing until two days after Lisa was born as a result of the medication I was taking (morphine to bring my blood pressure down). Once we were able to begin, there were a few more problems. Lisa slept most of

the time when she was with me, so I didn't get to practice very much. I was anxious to get home and out of the hospital. Once home, I relaxed; and the nursing became a special time, and an easy task. My mother helped out for the first three weeks. Although I never really felt my milk 'let down,' Lisa was content. Once my mother left I'm sure I tensed up as now I had sole responsibility all day every day. During this time, there was always the question in the back of my mind, 'Am I doing this right?' I think the initial problems affected me more psychologically than physically."

Some new mothers do not want their own mothers around; others (see the "Anthropology of the Mother's Mother," in Chapter VIII) do want their mothers there. In this instance, Mrs. Appleton felt a real loss when her mother left.

Mr. and Mrs. Appleton came in for a routine check-up when their daughter was fifteen months old. She was a smart, delightful little girl who would smile at me as long as she was next to her mother or father. Her father worked the night shift while her mother worked during the day, so one parent was with her at all times. Lisa was very attached to her parents. She had normal stranger anxiety and, every time that I came near her, she would shift closer to her mother, suck her right thumb, and reach back and twirl her mother's hair with her left hand.

I explained the origin of the "normal" trichotillomania (See "transitional objects" in the glossary) and that, in fact, she was attached to the mother's hair as a transitional object. To test this, I asked the mother to hold her in her arms while I slowly approached. The father instinctively and protectively came over. As I approached, to the surprise of us all, she not only reached out for her mother's hair but also simultaneously reached for her father's hair. Lisa was equally attached to both parents.

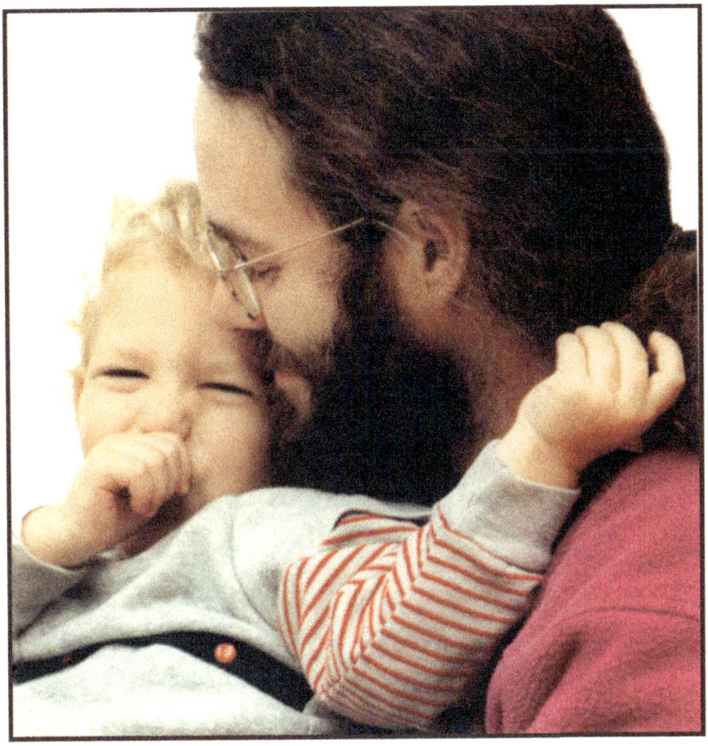

Normal Trichotillomania

The mother announced that she was pregnant and due in five months. She expressed anxiety about trying to breast-feed again. I brought up her letter of fifteen months ago. I pondered aloud about something I had wondered about for a long time. Was Mrs. Appleton ***actually*** *having difficulty separating (feeling the loss of) from her own mother?*

I wondered, together with Mrs. Appleton, if what happened before was possibly that she was fine and happily breast-feeding as long as her mother was around. But, when her mother left and Mrs. Appleton was alone, she had difficulty being successful and breast-feeding all on her own. I explained that separation was like a student going off to college for the first time and longing to come back home for that first

Thanksgiving vacation. Mrs. Appleton's face brightened, it was as if a light bulb had been turned on.

I left the room for an emergency. Upon return, Mr. and Mrs. Appleton were actively discussing the situation themselves.

Just as it was hard for Mrs. Appleton to separate from her mother, it was likewise difficult to help her own daughter to separate from her. For this reason, she had not encouraged a separate transitional object, even when I encouraged doing so earlier. The daughter's transitional object was attached to the parents' heads...their hair.

Their second child was delivered and named Megan. Again, Mrs. Appleton's mother visited to help-out. However, this time Mrs. Appleton encouraged her to stay for only a very short time. Mrs. Appleton's sister called and offered help. Mrs. Appleton expressed her gratitude for the offer but told her sister she wanted to do everything by herself this time. The breast-feeding was successful. Mrs. Appleton expressed joy over feeling less anxious and more in control of her own "stand independently" feelings.

Mrs. Appleton's mother came for another visit when Megan was six months old. She gave constant recommendations on childcare. Finally, Mrs. Appleton asked her husband in private, "I wonder what she thinks I do when she's not around?" He comforted her, "Don't worry, she'll be leaving on Thursday."

For some, approaching being successful creates feelings of anxiety and guilt followed by depression. Mrs. Appleton had such a wonderful mother. How could she ever match her or be better than her own mother? The story above illustrates why Mrs. Appleton failed to successfully breast-feed her first child; it was as if she wanted to unconsciously protect the dependent bond between herself and her own mother. To Mrs. Appleton, being a successful mother meant becoming independent of her own mother. That loss was fraught with fear and apprehension. Mrs. Appleton gained a beautiful baby girl, but she did not want to lose her own mother. She was not ready for this by herself: *"I tensed up as now I had sole responsibility all day every day."* These feelings undoubtedly contributed to her failure to breast-feed following her mother's departure after Lisa was born: *"During this time there was always the question in the back of my mind, 'Am I doing this right?'"* Mrs. Appleton wanted her mother back; she did not know what to do without her. When her mother left, her preoccupying anxiety inhibited her breast milk production; and she had to switch to formula. It was as if to be successful in breast-feeding would mean losing her own mother. So, when her mother left, the breast-feeding failed.

It is not uncommon for mothers, who have been raised usually in a "rescue" mode and who thus remain extremely dependent on their own mothers, to be understandably apprehensive about making their own decisions and doing things on their own. Breast-feeding is something that only a mother herself can do. While someone else may give advice, the ultimate task is the mother's alone.

For advice mothers may turn to professionals (nurses, lactation consultants, doulas) to help them sort out the initial difficulties of having a new infant. The need for these mentors to help the mother separate and stand on her own two feet should not be criticized; it is a healthy approach to childbearing. It should not be perceived as any different than having basketball, soccer, tennis, or golf lessons from a coach. But usually, unless a mother gains sufficient insight, the anxiety about losing the dependency on her own mother will not go away regardless of a lactation professional. (Also see "*Trying to Please Everyone but Not Harry.*")

> ***The tale of Mrs. Appleton and her mother goes on:***
> The Appletons recently came in, again for a routine exam. Mrs. Appleton reported at this office visit that her mother and sister had been visiting. Her mother wanted to take charge and toilet train both children, now one-year-old Megan and two-and-half-year-old Lisa. Mrs. Appleton disagreed with her mother. A rather vociferous argument

> ensued. It was interrupted when the older, unmarried sister of Mrs. Appleton walked in wondering, "What are you two arguing about?" Mrs. Appleton had her way. Her own mother left, totally flummoxed, not to mention a bit miffed. Mrs. Appleton explained, "I do not want my children to grow up as dependent upon their mother as I was!" It was interesting that during this examination Mrs. Appleton, for the first time, failed to "rescue" the children from me. She stood back, reassured them ("empathy"), but clearly expected them to handle their own fears. She appeared for the first time to be content, perhaps trusting enough to let them master their own worries. (See Rescue versus Empathy in Chapter XIII)

Many new mothers unconsciously fear/feel that to be successful as a mother sometimes may feel like they are irreversibly severing the tie with their own mothers. They perceive that as an unacceptable loss, as if it were the **Ultimate Loss**. Because that feeling can be unconsciously strong, some parents, like Mrs. Appleton in the above story with breast-feeding her first baby, are actually unable to be successful. This is called Success Neurosis. Depression and worry that it is *"all up to me, I'm on my own,"* can then descend, like a pall, upon a mother; and that as well can intensify a mother's inability to be successful. This Success Neurosis can also be one of the unconscious causes of postpartum depression. The dynamics and solution of the maternal success neurosis thus may come into conflict with the dynamics of "the Anthropology of the Mother's Mother."

To be successful should not necessarily mean that the relationship with the mother's mother is replaced or lost forever. But if a new mother is that dependent upon her own mother, it can feel like the Ultimate Loss. However, the tie need not be severed irreversibly. A new relationship can hopefully evolve between a grandmother and her daughter, who is now the new mother. They can become closer in a mentoring relationship and/or as mature adult friends.

But…that is a role that some of the mothers' mothers are very reluctant to accept. These grandmothers are often extraordinarily entrenched and unwilling to accept that they may need to give up, or rather change, their own role as mother in order to let their daughters thrive in their roles as new mothers. But it is hard, very hard, to feel as if you are not needed. All of this "rescue" and dependency usually comes from generations above, the Ghosts in the Nursery.

Now the following is a bit hard to actually report, and fathom, but it happens, and not so infrequently: Some grandmothers seem to promote dependency. And they can tie their children, as they grow up, to a very strong rope of dependency. It seems to keep the grandmother in a role of superiority and dominance, and important for being always needed. At times, it can seem that they want their child, now the new mother, to fail so that they, the grandmother, are then still needed to rescue them. These grandmothers seem to have an amazingly strong protective shell around their own sense of self; so much so that discussions of all of this can be threatening, *really threatening*, and create great apprehension in a new mother on how to deal with it, on how to if possible approach this with her own mother. If the grandmother is confronted with it she can, in fact, make you feel like you are trying to kill her, destroy her in her role. That grandmother can furiously protect herself and, in her rage, sometimes narcissistically reject her own daughter who is now trying to be a mother. She, feeling seemingly unneeded and truly wounded, can walk away from her own daughter! (See not only "*The Ultimate Loss Perceived*," above but also "*Hypnotic Suggestions and the Wildest of Dreams*" and "*The Carefree Socialite*," below) This happens, unfortunately way too often.

On the other hand, an increasing number of mothers have been raised by their own mothers to be independent. Upon becoming mothers, these women are less worried about becoming independent of their own mother, for they have been raised and encouraged from early childhood to feel good about their own independent accomplishments. They have learned as they grew up that independent actions were gratifying and that, indeed, they did not lose the actual relationship with their own now mother, a grandmother now quite proud of her daughter's accomplishments.

"I Will Not Repeat What My Parents Did to Me!"

The feelings described above highlight the apprehension about doing well that is felt by some parents who perceive their own parents as perfect role models. Others, however, may not have experienced what they consider to be good parenting. These parents may vow not to repeat what their parents did to them. They may wish frequently, or even constantly need, to place distance between themselves and their own parents to protect themselves and their children from the grandparents. Despite this, such parents are often amazed and chagrined at hearing themselves use the same phrases that they objected to when used by their own parents.

The Homunculus Phenomenon

Sometimes parents treat a newborn baby as if he were an adult. If a "high-strung" baby screams, some parents believe the baby is acting intentionally: *"He wants to act that way, he's being just plain mean." "He is not supposed to be acting that way." "He's possessed. I need an exorcist!"* The frustration of not being able to console one's infant can lead to anger toward the child without the parent being aware of its source.

It is during this time that many parents tell professionals that they can, for the first time, understand what leads to child abuse. In true infant abuse cases, the infant may be high-strung and have colic; and the parents, thinking the infant ought to behave, physically retaliate for the infant's apparent hostile act, as if he were intentionally misbehaving. The abusing parents do not have just a fantasy (as described in the preceding paragraph) but treat the infant as if he were truly a little adult, a homunculus. Thankfully, most parents recognize the fantasy as nothing more than that. They verbalize it to a spouse and feel relieved. They then are able to go back to warm caring.

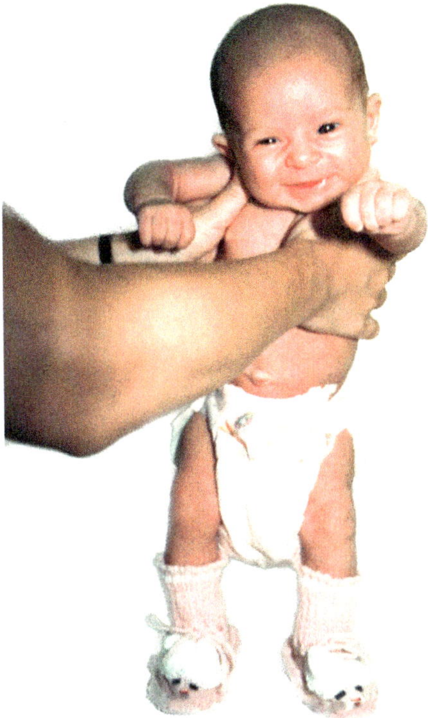

"I'm really not a homunculus! I'm just a little kid."

The Older Sibling(s)

Parents who already have a child usually have fewer worries and fears about success, unless they have been dealt a serious specific problem, such as multiple miscarriages or a special-needs first child. Most second-time parents are calmer about their new infant's frustrations. They allow the child to express himself with crying, worrying less that it will irrevocably ruin his personality.

A common apprehension, however, remains: *"How can I love someone else as much as I love this one?"* Worries grow about adjusting again to a new relationship, about becoming intimate with yet another new person. Preoccupying fears can develop in trying not to shortchange either the new baby or the older child. These worries may be renewed concerns about giving up more of one's self and successfully taking on yet another new role.

We are usually raised to be intimate with only one other person at a time. Yet, when children come along, we must become intimate with more than one individual at the same time. Parents, especially mothers, worry about how they will accomplish this. Those who grew up mastering on an everyday basis the relationships within a close family usually experience these conflicts less frequently.

If there is a one-and-a-half to two-year gap between the new infant and the older sibling, the older sibling is in the midst of the "first individuation." That means he is practicing being his own boss, an individual, but is still very attached to his parents and is very conflicted between independence and dependence. At this age, he will not have mastered his separation fears. He may be hard to get to sleep or he may renew waking at night, especially toward the end of the pregnancy. In the morning, he may scream until picked up by a parent. He may become terribly upset when the parents leave the room during the day. He will often regress and act younger. If he is toilet trained, he may start soiling. He may do many things to get his parents' attention, often setting up struggles like not wanting to put on his clothes in the morning. Such struggles can lead to a competition between parent and child about who is in control, who is the boss. A struggle leaves him in charge and the parents on a short leash. It's his way of being the boss and in control but not losing you; you are connected to the other end of the leash! It's his way of getting your attention, so you are looking at him and not the new infant. (Much, much more on this in Book IV)

The parents, feeling his fears and his dependence, wonder how they're going to manage this behavior along with caring for the new infant. They wonder and worry about how lonely and abandoned he may feel? If a parent works outside the home, the parent can feel additional guilt about being unavailable. The parent can feel that the older sibling will feel even more abandoned when the parents leave for work in the morning. "*This is tough; I am not there for anybody.*"

This may be an opportunity to grow. While the older sibling may feel alone and, perhaps, less loved, it is a time to teach: To teach the older sibling that though life has changed, he is nonetheless loved as much as before. He does not need to worry. Let him know these words: "*You have a place in my heart! It is just for you. And no one ever takes that place. You don't need to worry. I love you.*"

As an aside: If the first sibling is older (by, say, four years or more) and has begun to have a life of his own with cooperative play with his own friends, and is beyond the age of "first individuation," beyond the age of raw ego, then the conflicts with the new infant are far less. Not nonexistent, but far less. (More on this will appear in Chapter XIII of this book as well as in Book IV. But also see the actual photos of this in Book I.)

Worry

I have given up trying to stop parents from worrying. As mentioned before, worry comes with love. Once you love someone, you worry, and there is no way to escape that aspect of parenthood.

It is that simple...but not quite that simple. Worry can go beyond concern and become a preoccupying obsession. It can also flip into Guilt. Worry then evolves beyond simply worrying and goes for a wish to control outcomes, to protect, and make things better. But the reality is that despite all attempts, parents cannot control everything. That is a very hard pill to swallow (see "Wish versus Reality"). And when they can't control everything, worry can flip to guilt and guilt to magic, which is a whole other discussion to follow later in this book.

Does

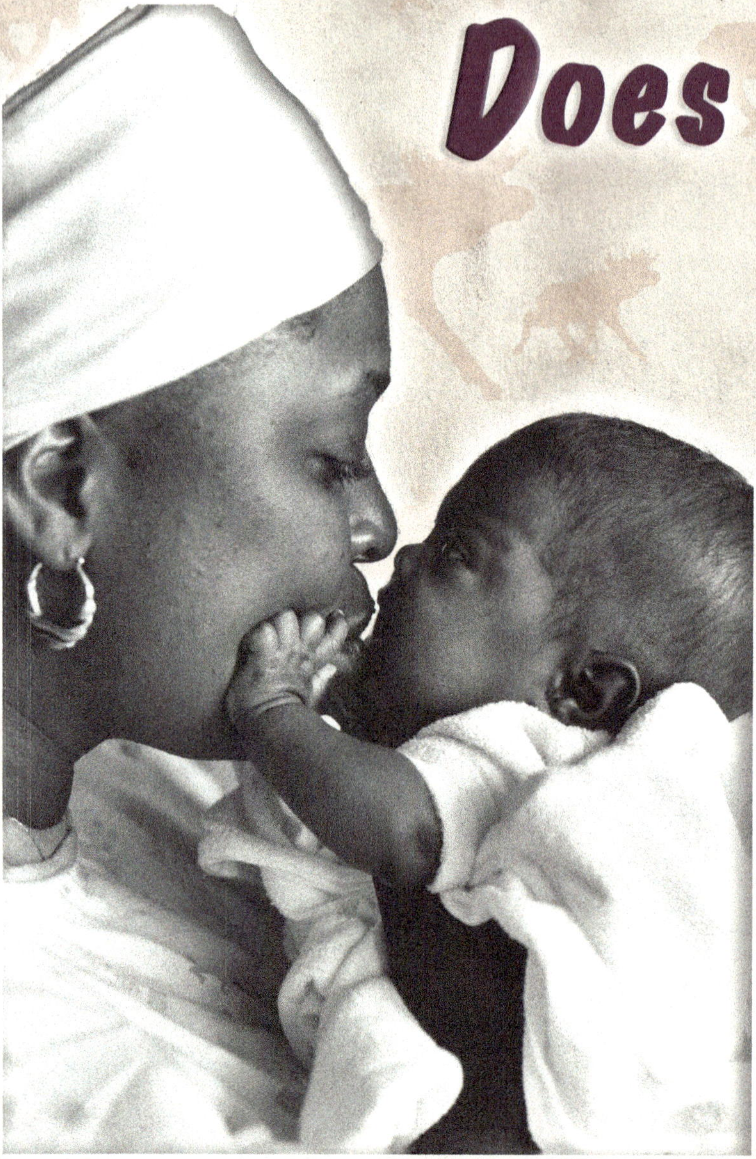

he know me?

Part II:
Does He Recognize Me?

What's

he

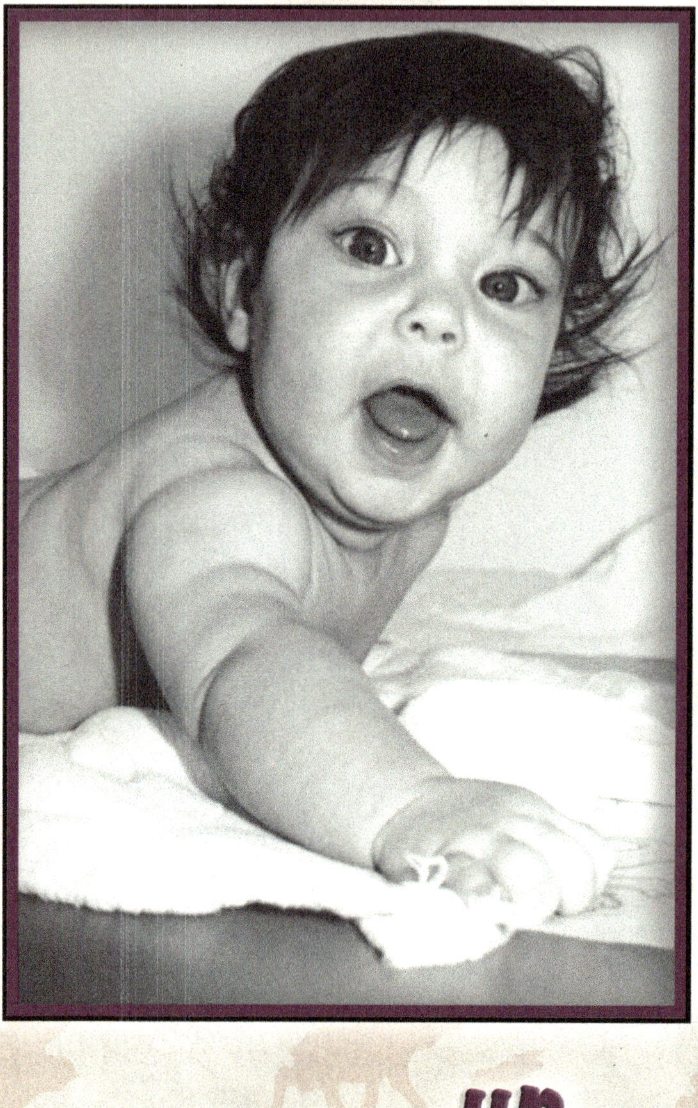

up

to?

Chapter V:
What Is He Up To?

From Reflex to Control...and Then Intention

When born, they come out with needs, reflexes, and their temperaments. It's that simple.

Ok, maybe a birthmark or two.

But, while a bit obvious, this is worth discussing so we know what to expect: Their needs are warmth and nutrition and cuddling closeness. So, we dress them and wrap them in wonderful outfits, or whatever we have. We feed them; and that has all its issues. And we cuddle with them; and that feels good to us as well. And then as we take care of their needs, as we water the flower, they grow and blossom.

But what grows and blossoms? Well, obviously, they grow in weight and height. So, first an interesting fact: They don't grow continuously; they grow in **spurts**. That explains why they may contentedly feed for a short bit of time but then suddenly want more for a day or two as they insist that supply catch up with the demand of their growth that has just suddenly happened.

But their brains also grow and develop. Initially, they are dominated by reflexes with a temperament that modulates those reflexes. The startle reflex, the grasp reflex, and the rooting reflex are examples of what are called infantile automatisms, or uncontrollable infantile reflexes. These are described in Book I.

Interesting fact: The newborn's brain is born with more nerve cells than you and I have. As they organize these "wires" in the brain, the unneeded nerves die off, since they go unused. As they organize the remaining activated nerves/wires, they gain control initially of the reflexes. This is fascinating to watch.

Their inborn temperament modulates this whole process. So, some have more control than others and can self-calm from the get-go. Others with the high-strung temperament cannot "auto-calm" initially and need, for example, swaddling to stop their irritating startle reflex.

From the get-go, the newborn can do very little for themselves. We must fulfill all their needs because their uncontrollable reflexes are there preventing them from doing anything intentionally.

But then watch them! It's kind of amazing!!

First, he **must** get control of that startle reflex. So, what he initially does is to hold his arms stiffly outward to just stop the startle. Then, when he gets that, he works on stability by accomplishing either or both the following: He, while on his back, will clinch his fists and hold them against his chest to keep them from popping out into a startle reflex; or he will take his elbows and push them back onto the changing table like the stabilizers on a backhoe. He does this so he can prevent the startle reflex's rocking from side to side causing its out-of-control scary feeling of falling.

Ok, and Whew... Now, when he has this startle reflex under some sort of control, he can then start attempting something he wants to do; and that is a social smile with you. And when that happens you melt. He keeps trying, but to do it he must control the irritating and distracting startle reflex. So, he will hold himself still to smile, start to smile, but (in the beginning) then forget to continue to control the startle reflex, and then frustratingly lose the smile. Erg!... But he keeps working and practicing and eventually he can control the reflex sufficiently to get out more intentional smiles. This takes on the average about six weeks.

His next social action comes with his attempted cooing, his actual responsive communicating with you, either with a smile or a complaint. Now that's fun; it's like he is talking to you. But again, watch carefully. He must stop the startle reflex from distracting him from his wish to intentionally coo. So initially he will start to coo, but then OMG forgets to prevent the distracting startle reflex. So, he goes after it again, and then again, as he practices cooing. It is just like learning a sport; it takes practice and practice before a smooth accomplishment.

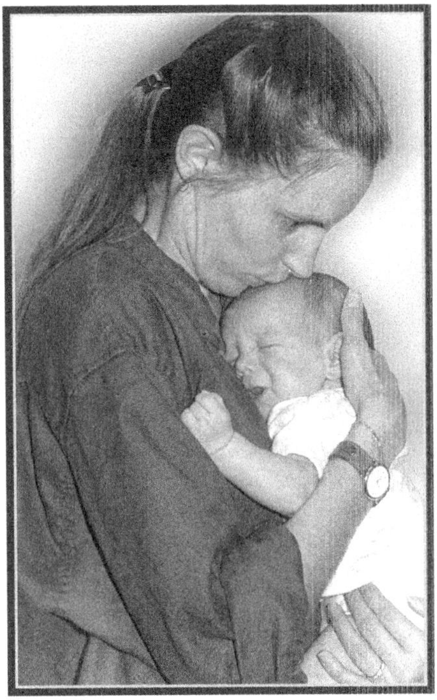

"It's ok; you're gonna get there."

Then he works on back support. But also, he works on control of his arms and hands. He has to learn to stop the grasp reflex before he can intentionally reach, touch, and get hold of something; so, he practices holding his hands open. And as the weeks go by he learns, as he dominates and stops his reflexes, to intentionally reach and touch and to do so softly without being forced by the grasp reflex to grab. **And then he intentionally touches you!**

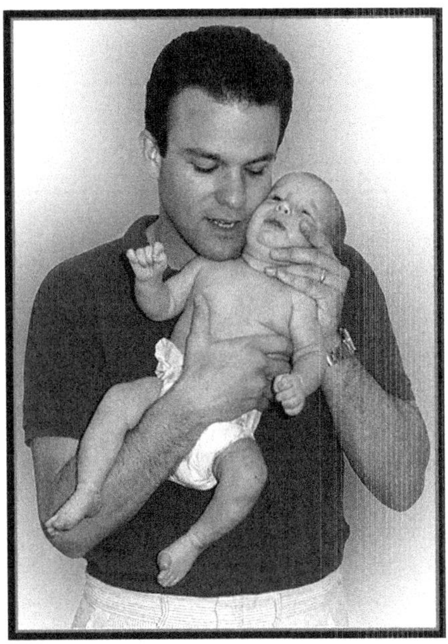

"Hang in there big guy! I'm with you."

It is really fun to watch! And I bring it up because that's when he recognizes you, and socially interacts with you, and eventually and intentionally touches and bonds more and more with you. This all happens in the early months. This is called the Homeostatic Period of development, the time when his wishful brain, always acting faster than his body, eventually seizes some control to then perform intentional acts. And as each petal opens you see his social and intellectual person exposed to your delight.

So, he goes from reflex to control to intention as he develops further tools for bonding and intimacy. It's awesome! It's pretty cool: especially that first smile, then the coo, and then that reaching out touching you. You melt, truly melt! You actually experience that hormonal upper from his gentle touch of your skin!

Nurture Needs

Sleep?

> ***Sleep?***
> *My daughter had an extended period of time when she was not sleeping well (to the extent that my husband and I started tracking on an app how many minutes she spent eating, sleeping, and "playing" / being alert). I would try to describe my frustrations to people: "She only slept eight hours yesterday!" People would cheer and congratulate me until I corrected them: NOT IN A ROW...TOTAL! They would be stunned into silence and mutter something about how quickly this magical time would pass ("stop complaining about sleepless nights because any minute she'll be off to college and you'll miss this..."). All advice disappeared. Other parents would stop talking to me (as though her sleeplessness was contagious). It was not until her four-month check-up when it was discovered she lost significant weight did it become obvious that she wasn't sleeping because she was not getting enough calories from nursing.*

Why are we discussing sleep? This book is part of *The Psychological Survival Guide for Parents* series and that has nothing to do with sleep, right? Well if they don't sleep, you don't sleep! And no sleep does not make for a happy parent, especially a parent who has to handle a lot of the changes and stresses that come with a new child. Lack of sleep for you lowers your tolerance, makes you cranky at best! Also, most of the sleep problems come about from the concepts we are discussing in this series such as "Rescue versus Empathy" and "*I don't want you to ever feel like I felt.*" For now, hang in there. We will discuss how and why problems occur and how to prevent them in this book's Part IV, which deals with coping concepts. But to know what to expect, it's a good idea to realize what is normal. And we'll discuss that here.

The First Three days

Often after delivery, a newborn is exhausted and will sleep quite a bit.

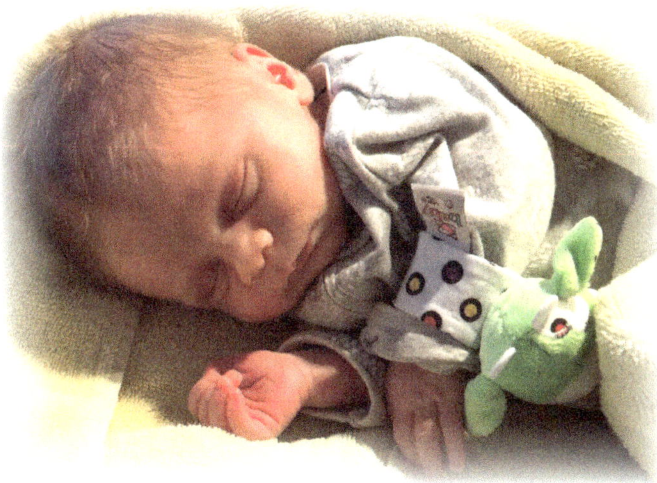

"Wow, he's pretty nice."

If all is normal, they are often not interested in nursing or taking much formula for the first three days or so. Why? Well, what happens is that during pregnancy they store up calories and fluids. That is their way of protecting themselves until breast milk comes in on day three. So, they are not really hungry as they use up their stores during those first days. That's the way nature takes care of them; that's the way it was before formula existed. So, assuming no complications such as prematurity, they need nothing during those first days because they have the stores of calories and fluids already on board. And that is why all babies, even formula-fed babies, lose weight in the first days. So, while they are not hungry, they sleep a lot. (However, premature babies or babies that may have a low blood sugar may need something during this time. Thus, parents need to be flexible under those circumstances.)

The Early Weeks and Months, and Temperament

Newborns and infants in the early weeks have no circadian (circadian means daily, or 24-hour) sleep rhythms. It is truly as if they have jet lag from the nine-month trip in the dark no-sunshine womb. After they come out with birth they must now adapt to a big time-zone difference with astonishing daylight now added. **Consequently, a sleeping pattern that responds to this daylight does not develop and is not obvious until around one to three months of age.**

Before that they sleep a lot, usually around 16–17 hours total in a 24-hour day, depending on temperament. So, after the first three days, they sleep for 2–4 hours; they wake and want to feed, but then will sleep again. Hence, they will, with sleeping in between breast-feedings, wake to feed perhaps around 8–12 times within a 24-hour day. If formula-fed they will, more often than not, feed every 3–4 hours while sleeping in between feedings, thus wanting around only 6 or so feedings per 24 hours. By about 1–3 months they will **consolidate** their sleep (now getting over the jet-lag from the trip in the dark womb) usually at night as they adapt to daylight.

But then you need to ask yourself what you would prefer: If you put them down at 9 p.m., they will wake up at ~3 a.m. wanting to feed. But if you wake them and then tank them up at, say, 11 p.m., they will arouse around 5–6 a.m. Most, I think, would rather wake them to feed at 11 p.m. so all can sleep a bit later in the early morning.

Somewhere between 2–5 months they will regulate themselves to sleep not only at night but will also consolidate their sleep to a morning and afternoon nap during the day. Life for you then becomes more predictable and under your control... sort of. (See Chapter XI for enhancing their sleep and avoiding usual pitfalls.)

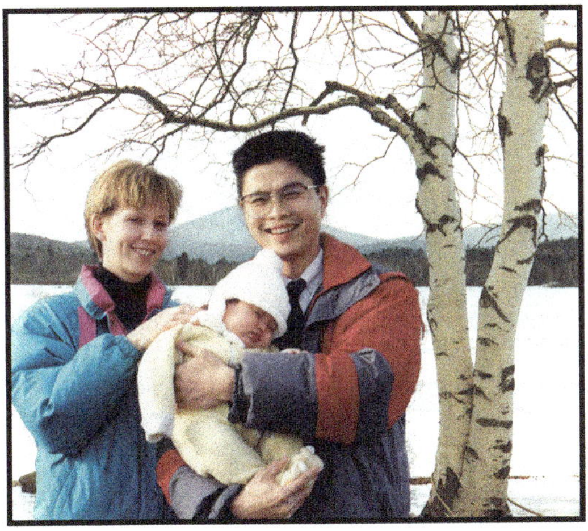

"I'm telling you: When it's nap time, he'll sleep anywhere."

Infants with high-strung temperaments sleep less than mellow kids. They have more sleep problems as well. They require more swaddling, and for more months. Why? Well, they can't control their startle reflex; and that infuriates them. As a mellow infant goes to sleep you can see them twitch slightly before relaxing further down into a deeper sleep. (Many adults do this as they go from the light phase of sleep into deeper sleep; these twitches are called "myoclonic jerks" and are part of initiating normal sleep.) But this twitching in the high-stung infant, who is unable yet to control his reflexes, suddenly evokes the startle reflex, which then jerks him awake. He is now furious at being awoken and no longer able to easily go back to sleep (thus no initial auto-calming is part of the high-strung temperament). So, then what happens is that you walk them around and/or feed to help them back to the beginning of sleep. You then try to put them down just after they fall asleep.

But the problem with that is that, as they hit the mattress while still in that light beginning phase of sleep, they startle and become ragingly awake again. **That is why they are or need to be swaddled** (see Book I for technique), **and swaddled well.**

Some parents find it easier to put the high-strung infants asleep on their tummies because then their hands and arms are against the mattress protecting them from going into a full-blown startle reflex: if on their backs, the hands and arms are free to go up and around into a full startle reflex.

But as some say, *"Back to sleep, tummy to play!"* And why? Why do they say that? It is well established that sleeping on the back prevents Sudden Infant Death Syndrome. So, wisest is to swaddle and having them sleep on their backs! And you can keep swaddling up until the brain dominates and controls the reflexes at around 3½ months of age or so when homeostasis is developed. However, most will continue to swaddle beyond that because without it the twitching will awaken the rage-inducing startle reflex even beyond that time. Most parents with a high-strung infant will, in fact, continue to swaddle until around a year of age. Just one more reason why it helps to recognize temperament early on!

How Breasts Work

"He just got delivered. Doesn't he need to be fed?"

"And what is happening to my breasts in these first few days?"

With delivery, and particularly with the delivery of the placenta, a trigger takes place to bring in milk on day three. During pregnancy, the breasts grew as they were being primed to make milk. But with the delivery of the placenta, the trigger is pulled. No matter what happens the milk will come in. You can sleep for three days, and the milk will still come in. Even if your baby may have been taken to the intensive care nursery away from you, the milk will still come in. So, you do not need to worry but you do have to wait until around day 3. Milk will come in.

You can use those first few days of no-milk-coming-out to practice the three breast-feeding positions: the cross-cradle, the football, and the side-by-side position. Learning those positions and rotating through them helps avoid sore, cracked nipples. The rotation changes the sucking pressure points around the nipple and evenly distributes them on the areola/nipple. If you use as often happens only one position, sore cracks may develop on each breast on the diagonal from his mouth always sucking in the same position. (See graphic of cracked nipples in Chapter XI. Google "Breast-feeding positions" to see illustrations of how to get into these positions.)

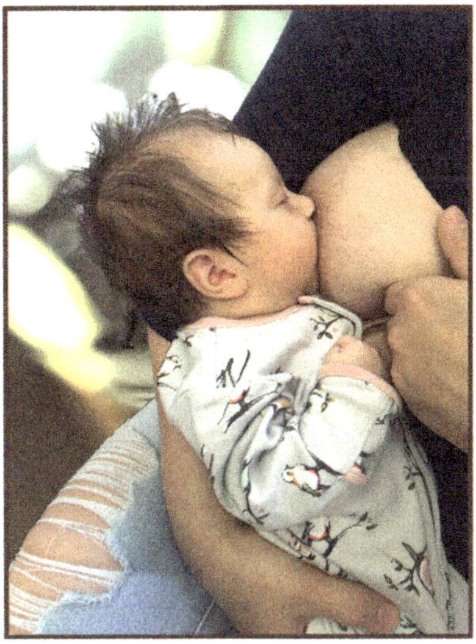

This is the "cradle" position. It is to be used only after your baby has already learned to breast-feed.

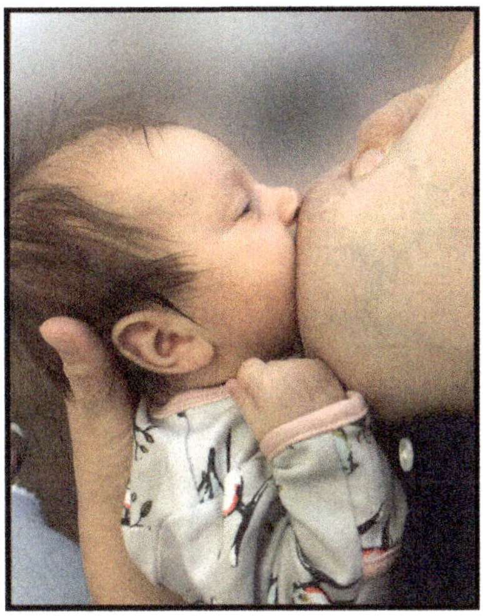

This is the "cross-cradle" position. Notice your hand behind and firmly holding his head guiding him to the nipple/areola. (see Book I for details). This is the best position for his learning to breast-feed. With your hand on the back of his head, you can guide him to latch on.

Those first few days can also be used to practice his latching onto the breast. But he may be both tired and satiated with the calories he already stored up during the pregnancy. He may not really even want to attempt latching on until he becomes hungry. (Lots of books and information are out there on all this.)

But then, while delivery triggers milk production, only one stimulus keeps it up! And **understanding this process will significantly help toward**

successful breast-feeding. That stimulus is the initiation of suckling (words chosen carefully). **It is not the longevity of suckling; it is the individual initiations of suckling** that are the only stimuli for continued milk production.

When the baby attaches to the nipple, a stimulus goes through the nerves from the nipple to around the chest wall to the nerves of the spinal cord and from there up to the top of the brain, and then down to the pituitary gland at the base of the brain. That stimulus forces that gland to release into the blood a pulse of two hormones, oxytocin and prolactin. Traveling in the blood, prolactin goes to the breast tissue and says, "Make milk." Oxytocin goes to microscopic cuffs of muscle tissue around the ducts of every gland in the breast and forces a contraction of that tissue, which in turn milks the milk out. That is called the "let down," now known as the "milk ejection reflex." Thus again, it is **not the longevity** of breast-feeding that brings in more milk; **it is the frequency**.

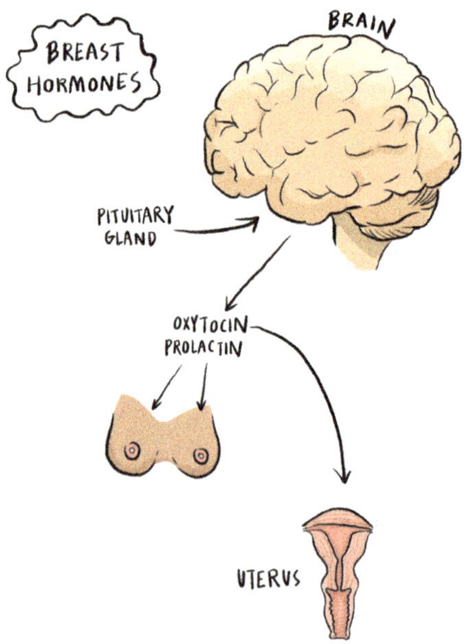

Now another factoid, which is not insignificant: **most of the breast milk initiated by the pulse of hormones comes out in the first minutes** (see the graph). You do not need to breast-feed for more than 8–10 minutes per side. You can also give 2–4 minute per side snacks to stimulate more milk production, and he still gets a significant amount of the milk from your breasts (see the graph). Hence, the more frequent the initiations of suckling, the more pulses of prolactin (and oxytocin), and thus more milk is produced.

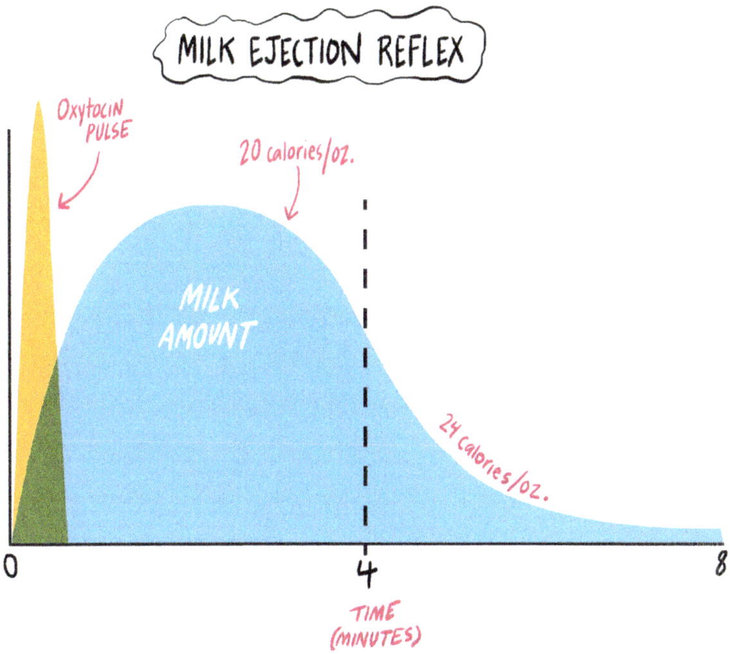

Midnight Crying

One mother called me around midnight sobbing with tears that she had been breast-feeding continuously since noon, twelve hours ago, and her baby was still screaming with hunger. She cried he was getting nothing from her! She was beside herself! And she was right: he was getting nothing at this twelfth hour of continuous breast-feeding. The breasts had mainly been

> *stimulated once to make milk; and that was at noon when she initiated the feeding. (More prolactin and oxytocin pulses can come out with continuous breast-feeding, but nothing like that initial pulse.)*

Frequent brief breast-feedings are far better than infrequent long breast-feedings. Why talk about this? Well, if all of this is moving forward to working well, then baby and family will be happier!

Some will offer advice: *"Just let him feed as long as he wants."* Well...some babies have a strong sucking need that is not actually a hunger need. And if you let them use you as a pacifier, you will end up with sore cracked nipples; and soon there is little enjoyment of this wonderful child. So again, "**frequent brief breast-feedings are far better than infrequent long breast-feedings**."

The breast milk that comes out in the initial minutes is about 20 calories per ounce; after that it is less in quantity but around 24 calories per ounce. That latter part of the ejected milk some will call the "rich hind" milk. But there is not much of that in quantity after about 8 minutes of suckling on that side. Long breast-feedings are not only unnecessary but will, in fact, end up with less milk production, and with painfully sore, cracked nipples. More on all of this in the Coping Concepts of this book. (See the figure of the Milk Ejection Reflex.)

Book I also has photos of the different positions for latching on and breast-feeding, and discusses breast-feeding the high-strung infant. Temperament and breast-feeding is an issue; and that is discussed in Book I. And, of course, "breast feelings" are an issue.

THE INTIMACY DRIVE

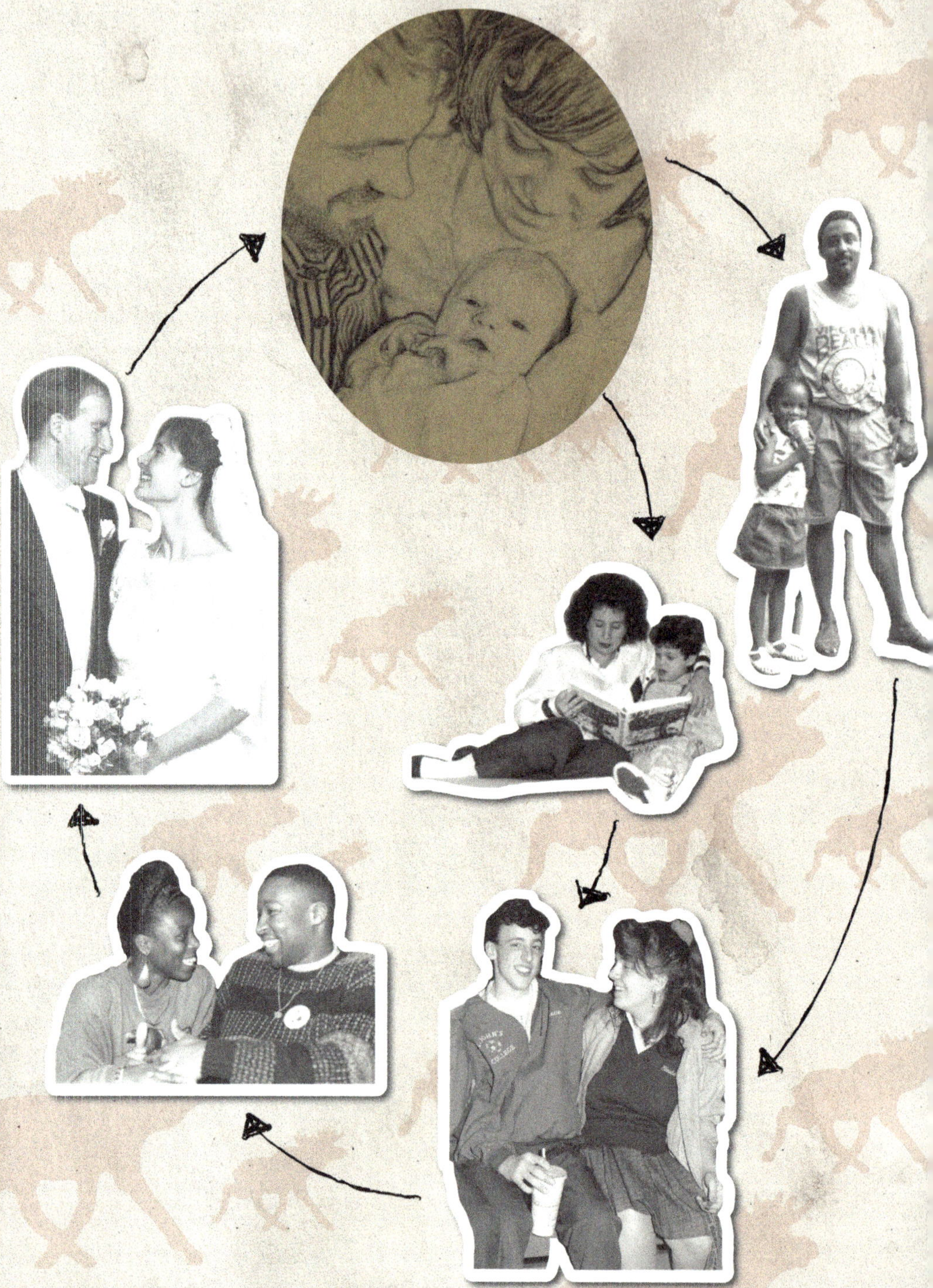

Chapter VI:
The Intimacy Drive

"Will I love him? Will he love me?"

On the Radio

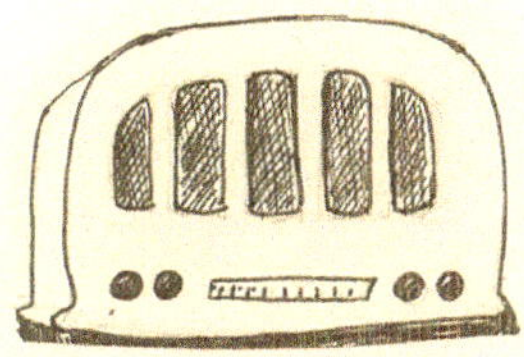

Years ago, on the radio, a talk-show host the late Ann Landers invited mothers to call or write in to express whether they enjoyed the experience of having a baby enough to do it again. Astoundingly, two thirds of mothers who responded indicated they were not interested in repeating the experience.

My impression is that most mothers I have known would respond differently. Clearly, Ann Landers's survey was not a statistically valid approach. Perhaps those who responded wanted to express their strong, negative feelings, while those with a positive experience, feeling they had no "cross to bear," did not respond. More significantly, most mothers go on to have more than one child (The Chicago Tribune said in 1991 that about 80 percent of Americans have at least one sibling).

But Ann Landers's survey highlights a serious point. A weighty proportion of mothers are less than thrilled with delivering a baby and their motherhood that follows. Many mothers enjoy their child as an infant and, indeed, are sad to see him/her grow older. Others are vexed and not always enthralled with their newborn.

Addressing this vexation is one of the goals of this book: increasing parental knowledge of the psychological development of parents, along with the physical and psychological development of the child. My hope is that, with heightened awareness, quality experiences will enhance parent-parent and parent-child relationships as well as reduce anxiety, thus resulting in a flourishing of The Intimacy Drive!

Attachment

A Process, Not an Event

Is there an actual Intimacy Drive?

I think so. I think it appears as an ever-evolving circular drama of life with spheres of recurrent bonding:

Soon-to-be partners meet, they date, they talk and share, they touch, and they bond to each other. They have a child, and the infant and parents are driven toward seeking intimacy with each other. The infant separates from the parents, grows to maturity, and repeats the cycle of developing intimacy.

This Intimacy Drive is influenced by many factors, in particular the interaction between parent-to-parent and parent-to-infant temperaments. It is also impacted by the degree of support from relatives and friends. At the same time, the Intimacy Drive is constantly challenged by the earlier described Intruder Complex, sibling rivalry, and the need for any member of the mother/father/partner/infant triad to maintain a sense of self in the process.

Many parents are falsely told that, if they are unable to hold or breast-feed their infant immediately after delivery, bonding may not be as strong as it could be. This has been proven to be untrue. Many times a complication after delivery leads the child to be whisked to a special or intensive care hospital nursery; the parents and newborn may miss each other right after delivery.

Attachment is an enormously strong process that can withstand vehement pressures. Surviving a difficult experience can actually enhance bonding. Parents attach to formula-fed infants and tube-fed premature babies in incubators. Adopted children and parents bond. The attachment process is not fragile.

While pregnancy and the early months of life are indeed a very important period, bonding progresses over the lifetime of the child and parents. Only severe psychological or physical cataclysms can prevent the bonding process, and even then, its imagined presence is longed for.

It Goes Both Ways

During pregnancy, most parents long for the infant. The infant, while in the uterus, responds with a "kick" to let the parents know that he's really there. During the first weeks after delivery, he snuggles and the parents reciprocally seek that cuddling and eye contact. Parents feel a thrill, a rush, when they have the time to simply cuddle, skin-to-skin, with the newborn. It is a "rush!" Parents need and long for attachment just as much as infants do.

The Imprint for Adult Intimacy

Parents feel the drive and the desire for intimacy, closeness, love, and attachment with their new infant. This drive for physical closeness, mutual recognition, and firm attachment is presumed to be the pattern for adult intimacy. The drive is expressed in the rapturous quest for eye contact and recognition through sensual interactions involving vision, hearing, smell, and snugly, soft, secure embraces.

Parents wait agonizingly for the newborn's first smile. When it comes, much of the burden from the early weeks is forgotten. After that initial smile, the infant seeks the parents' recognition and social interaction begins. If ignored, the infant will often fuss until he can engage his parents in cooing conversation. Initially he will smile and coo with anyone. Within weeks, however, he becomes more familiar with his parents.

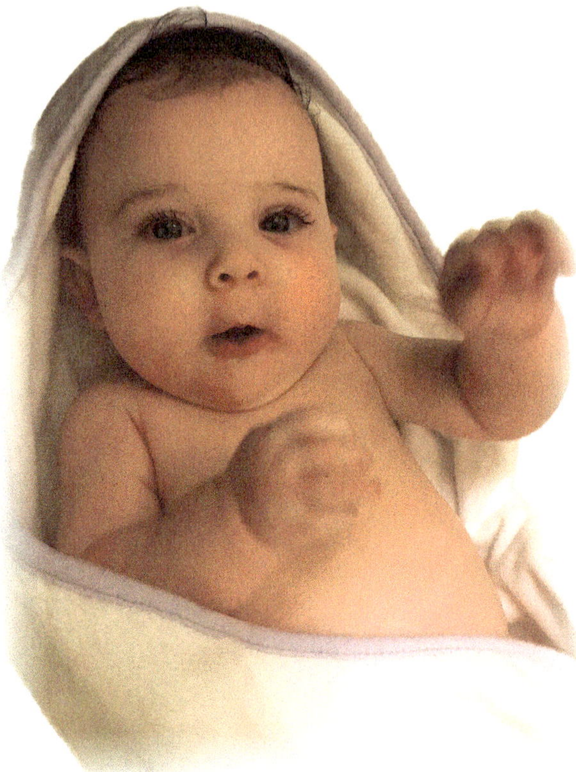

"You're sooo cute."

How deeply this drive is felt and fulfilled in infancy and throughout the first years of life plays a crucial role in determining his intimacy drive toward others when he becomes an adult. He then, in turn, bonds to a mate, and then he and his mate, in turn, bond to new offspring. If for whatever reason he is deprived of that bonding as an infant to a parent, he may bond to himself and become narcissistic as an adult.

So, do I think there is an Intimacy Drive?

Yep, I actually think it is true. And I actually also think we have a drive to be intimate, and therefore not alone. Moreover, I think there is a hormonal basis for it.

The Biochemistry of Love, and Bonding

Ok, hold onto your hats! This may sound a bit weird but it is fact.

Suddenly out of the clear blue sky on January 7, 1983, a research article appeared in the prestigious world-renowned journal *Science*. No explanation was given as to why it was accepted for publication in *Science*, as opposed to some journal of animal husbandry. It was just dropped in there among all these other unrelated highly scientific papers in the magazine. Its title: *Vaginal Stimulation: An Important Determinant in Maternal Bonding in Sheep.*

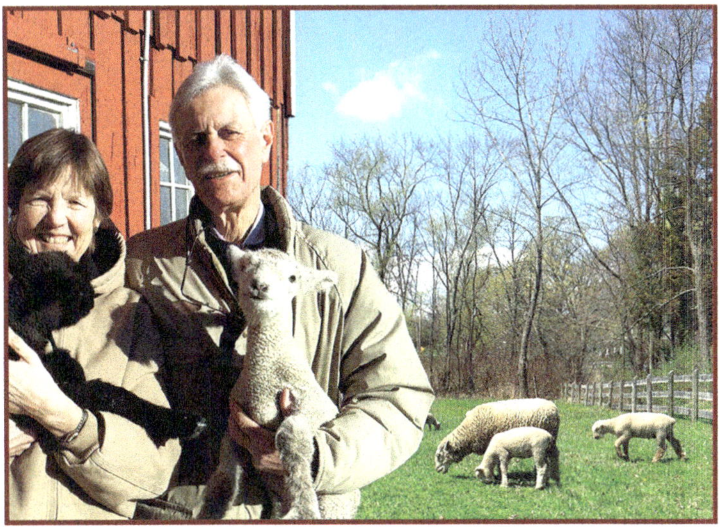

Dooo Ewe think she'lllll aaacept ussss ?

What they found was that an ewe would reject an alien lamb introduced into her own litter; it was obviously not hers. But if she were vaginally stimulated as the lamb was introduced she would accept and bond to that lamb as if it were part of her own litter! That scientific paper sparked a cascade of research into the biochemical aspects of bonding and love.

They found that the vaginal stimulation of the ewe induced oxytocin and that it was the oxytocin that promoted the bonding. It now appears that other neurobiological and endocrinological mechanisms are involved, but at the heart of these systems is the neuropeptide called oxytocin. Some even call it the "Love Hormone." Oxytocin ejects milk from the breast, contracts the uterus for delivering the baby. It is involved in maternal and probably paternal bonding, response to touch and goosebumps' induction, care-taking and protective aggression, the development of social bonds, stress responses and calming, and yearning and sexual arousal and orgasms. It is obviously not the only hormone involved in these processes. Endogenous opioids, dopamine, and vasopressin are other partners. But it is the major hormone in all of these social interactions.

Oxytocin's other actions explain:

- Why some mothers feel a uterine cramp, like a bad menstrual cramp, about 45 seconds after the baby attaches to the nipple during the first few days after delivery. (When the baby is put to the breast, oxytocin is stimulated and tells the breasts to eject the milk. But the oxytocin circulating in the blood after its release from the brain's pituitary gland also then forcefully contracts the muscle tissue of the uterus helping it to get back to normal size. See the figure on Breast Hormones.)
- Why a mother's breast will leak on the side opposite that being suckled.
- Why a mother may get vaginal wetness with a mini-orgasm when nursing.
- Why a mother's breasts may leak when she hears her baby cry, even from afar.

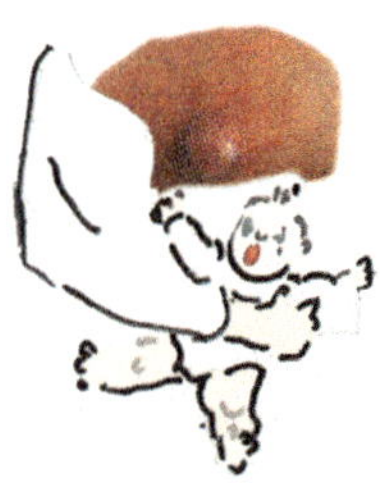

- And why her nipples become erect and her breasts leak, or even squirt, during love-making with her partner.

The glue of bonding is usually touch. A smell, a sound, a sight, or a presence can also evoke that feeling. That feeling can be in your gut, or tingle your skin, or cause sexual arousal or yearning. It is hard to put your finger on it or describe it; it is just felt. Perhaps it is best described, heard, and felt with poetry and song... the gist of bards.

All those feelings and occurrences are normal responses to the stimulation and release of oxytocin. A bonding hormone! Pretty amazing!

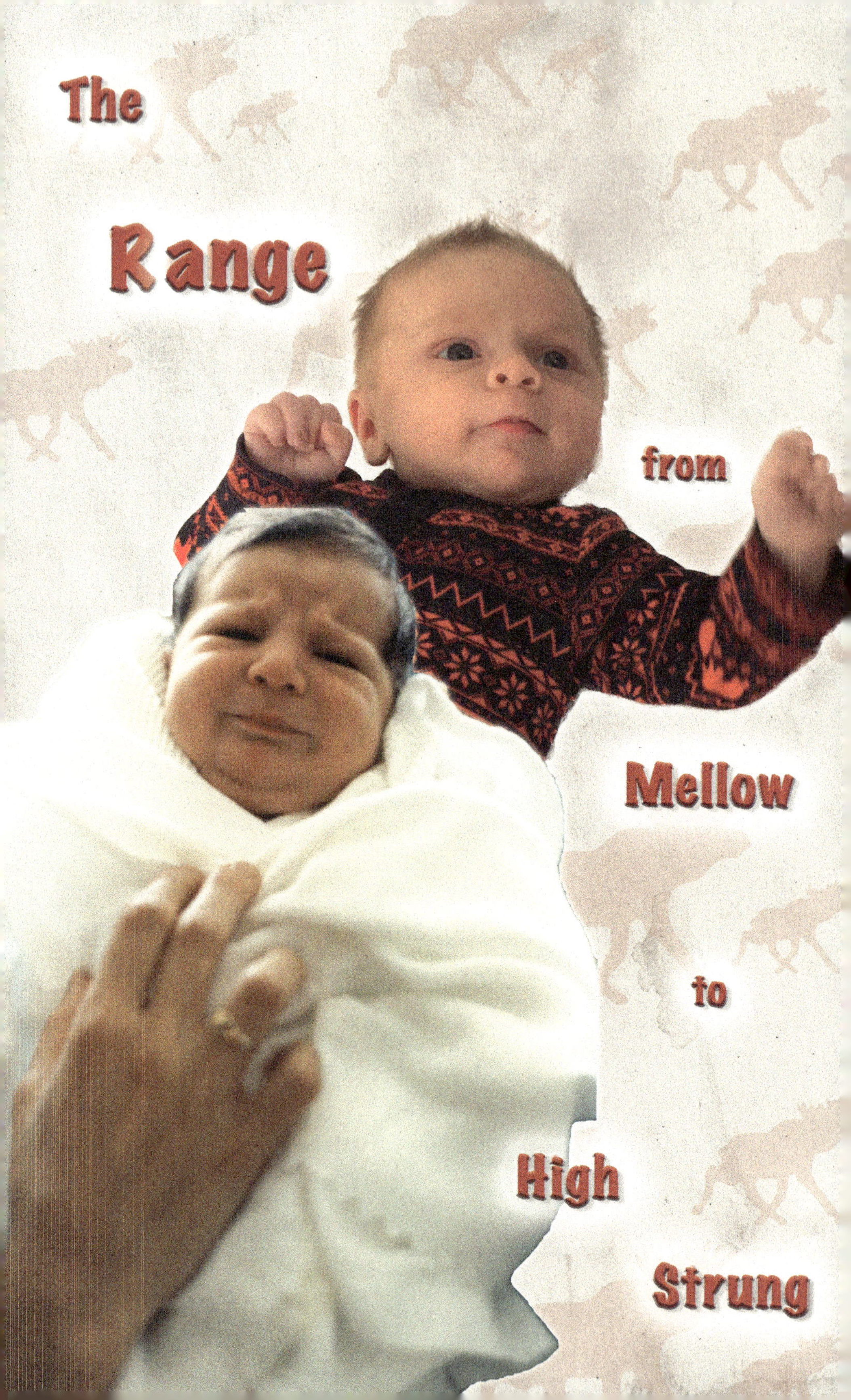
The
Range
from
Mellow
to
High
Strung

Chapter VII: Infant Temperament

Intimacy and Temperament

Matching and Mismatching

Temperament influences the Intimacy Drive. A parent(s)-to-be may be dreaming of and yearning for a warm, snuggly little baby but then receive a high-strung, reflex-dominated newborn capable of snuggling only when swaddled or during deep sleep. This can result in a "mismatching" and mismatching with its disappointing fears and anger can challenge bonding. But bonding will take place. In fact, it can at times drive the bond tighter because of the neediness for intense calming given the initial lack in the infant's self-calming ability. So, it is not always easy under those circumstances.

The Sometimes, Seeming Rejection by The Infant

Newborns look beyond us at the whole spectrum of their environment. They may ignore our eyes and look at all aspects of the periphery around our heads. This early lack of eye contact can feel like a rejection of our best efforts to engage with them. An understanding of this phenomenon helps parents accept the newborn's sometimes curious but indiscriminately insensate behavior.

Mismatches

The joyful parent is one that dreamed during pregnancy for a mellow cuddly newborn and actually received one. On the other hand, if a parent who wished for that mellow, cuddly newborn instead receives one that is high-strung, a conflict between the parent's wishes and the reality of the infant's temperament can be painfully felt (See "Wish vs. Reality" in Chapter XIII). A serious "mismatch" may then ensue when a parent, who is not aware of and does not appreciate the beauty of temperament variations, receives a high-strung newborn. The infant's apparent unhappiness undermines the mother and father's confidence. They wonder, "*What are we doing wrong?*" and sometimes anxiously question whether having a baby was worthwhile in the first place.

Making matters worse, in some cases, parents in this situation lack the knowledge or experience to cope with and calm the "high-strung" infant. If parents are informed about the good qualities of the different temperaments, they are at least prepared and can constructively help their high-strung infant adjust. They will eventually be thrilled with both his acquisition of skills and their own accomplishments. (See the anecdote: *The Carefree Socialite*)

Mismatches can also occur in the reverse scenario. One mother, a high-powered executive, received a beautiful, mellow, cuddly little girl. This mother was disappointed that she had not gotten a feisty "live-wire" with whom she could identify. A mismatch can be more than initially upsetting; it can also be a conflict for bonding, resulting in later psychological problems.

If parents watch their feelings carefully, they will notice that at first, they strive to do everything to make the high-strung infant happy. But at some point, all of these efforts fail. It is as if their baby is angrily rejecting their best efforts. These parents feel failure. These parents may become furious with the infant, sometimes fantasizing causing harm when they perceive the newborn infant as if he were a hostile adult rejecting their overtures. (See "Homunculus Phenomenon.") One father confessed, "*I thought he had a mean streak.*" Anger then quickly becomes replaced with guilt, sometimes resulting in a heavy parental depression.

It is helpful to realize that the high-strung baby's intermittent inconsolability is a variation of newborn temperament and that the negative points will melt away as the delightful aspects of his temperament emerge. This newborn has no innate wish to make his parents upset. This reflex behavior is not voluntary; he does not like it any more than his parents do. In fact, that is what makes him furious. It is not a failure of the parents; it is developmental. The cortex of the child's brain has simply not yet obtained dominance over those perplexingly rude newborn reflexes.

It is also helpful to realize that **"all anger is fear-based."** So, behind your anger may be a fear that you will not love him, or he will not love you, or a fear that your wish for a cuddly baby was thwarted. You might have the same temperament with its share of "frustration intolerance." So, to then identify with him/her may actually help.

It's Hard Being a Little Kid

Think about it. If he has an itch, he can't scratch it; he can't even tell someone where it is so they can scratch it! When irritated, all he can do is holler and hope...hope that you his parents can figure out the cause.

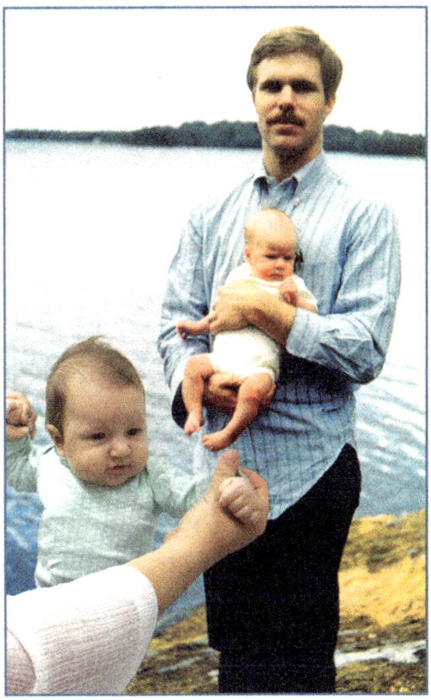

"Wow! It's a cool world out there!"

At the same time, the little kid also makes it difficult for us in the early weeks to feel that he, our newborn infant, is grateful. We want intimacy, and our new child may at times appear seemingly resistant.

But think about it again. Imagine what it's like for a newborn. For him, everything is surprise; he has just landed on a totally new planet. That is, in fact, quite true!!

Everything is so astonishingly new! While you are searching for eye contact he may look beyond you. I have always imagined it as growing up in the deciduous and fir forest of the northeastern United States and then flying to Arizona. As one disembarks from the plane in Tucson and looks about, one suddenly realizes, as dry warmth with its smells envelops you, that this is a strange, different, new world, a sea of desert and cactus, and new hues of light. This newborn has landed in a world of light and color and smells and sounds outside the dark, muffled womb. All is surprise and he startlingly looks beyond you, awed by this new world around and in front of him. Just watch his awe!

The newborn is tired after delivery. But relatively quickly he awakens. His needs and newborn reflexes become apparent and, soon thereafter, dominate. Hunger, warmth, and closeness are his needs. It is as if he longs to be back as a cub in the snuggly warm bear cave of the womb. His most obvious reflexes are the rooting, sucking, startle, and grasp reflexes. These reflexes, even when modulated by his temperament, may infuriatingly jerk him about and out of control; he hates that. This is especially true of the startle reflex for the high-strung infant. (See Book I for more details about infant temperament and reflexes.)

In the first few weeks and months he strives to gain control over his newborn reflexes. Once he masters them he can perform purposeful movements. Only then can he calm himself; only then can he express intentional signs of endearment, such as smiling and cooing followed by reaching, touching, and grabbing. And only then is he capable of accomplishing the beginnings of his drive toward intimacy with his parents.

A newborn may demand and cry to have his needs met while often giving little in return. He is not socially responsive other than with signals of complaint such as whimpers, cries, or screams. But **he is capable of interaction.** A newborn can certainly express emotion; it is usually unhappiness, discontent, or the quiet gratification of comfort. While he may feel content at times during the early weeks, he usually does not smile or socially interact with anyone. But he does recognize that something has been done in response to his demands. He does have emotional responses to his parents. He can curl his lower lip down far enough to break a parent's heart. He is, more often than not, consolable. As noted previously, all of these responses are modulated by his genetic temperament.

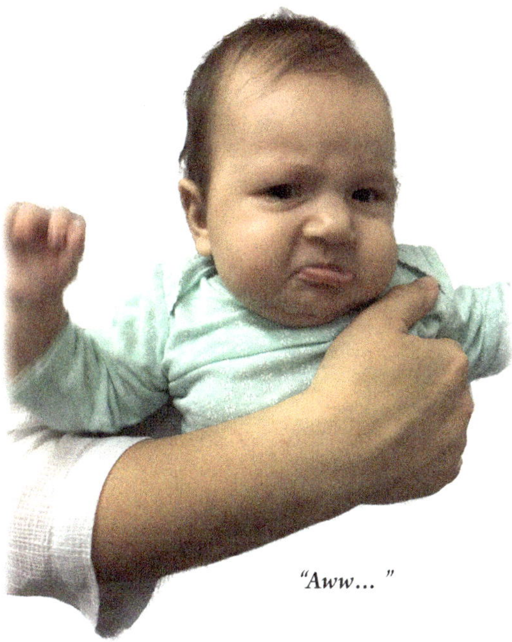

"Aww... "

His cries, with time, become discernible: Some are pouts with the lip curled out. Others are demanding expressions of hunger. Still others express hurt or discomfort. Often the cry of the high-strung newborn is absolute fury when faced with frustration. It is hard, **really hard, for new parents** to realize that the truly furious expression of frustration by the high-strung newborn is not deep unhappiness nor pain but rather a truly intense expression of frustration in a little body that knows no other way to express itself, like talking. He can't talk. He is actually just sticking up for himself! What's really great about this is that it is actually a quite cognitive process: His brain is working well, very well in his demanding fury! We just have to hang in there and with time, a long time, teach him how to express himself in more socially acceptable ways. That's our job. He's not just here for us; we are there for him. Over time, we parents recognize the different types of cries. But this indeed does take time; for new parents, it is usually weeks to a few months.

The Spectrum of the Great Modulator, Temperament

An individual newborn's temperament—or for that matter a child's or an adult's temperament—modulates the level at which he senses stimuli, expresses himself, and controls his reflexes and activity level. In the beginning, certain aspects of temperament are completely genetic. As a child grows, temperament is importantly molded by nurture.

Some newborns have more control over their irritations, expressions, and reflexes than others. For example, they are able to move their extremities more smoothly, even to the extent of being able to suck on their fingers or thumbs soon after birth, and sometimes even *in utero* (as seen on a sonogram). These infants have a "mellow" temperament. (The temperament researchers have other titles for different temperaments. But for simplification we will use a spectrum from the mellow to the high-strung.)

Sometimes just after birth, especially in an infant with a mellow temperament, the beginnings of social responsiveness can be seen and felt when eye contact is obtained. The infant can be consoled with a soft, understanding voice. Occasionally, in the immediate newborn period he can actually smile in response to endearing sounds. More often, though, the mellow newborn is rewarding to his parents by being content and easily consolable.

Infants at the other end of the spectrum of disposition have little control over their newborn reflexes. Being jerked out of control by the startle reflex can infuriate them. These high-strung newborns are hypersensitive, hyperreflexive, frustration-intolerant, and unable to calm themselves. They have the disconcerting task during these early weeks of mastering control over their reflexes to sufficiently calm themselves down. Only then can they go on to purposeful movements. (See Book I for more information about infant temperament and for a scale, the **TENP** (Temperament Evaluation of the Newborn by Peebles), which helps you determine your early infant's temperament type.)

When capable of purpose, the infant demonstrates his first non-reflexive, purposeful movement with a smile. At two to three months of age he begins cooing, having developed even more dominance over his newborn reflexes as the cortex of his brain develops.

Variations exist in the spectrum between the totally "mellow" and the totally "high-strung" newborn. Some babies will have a very strong temper and clearly demonstrate a will of their own. They have a very angry cry and arch their backs furiously out of control, as compared to the gentle compliant cry of the mellow newborn. It is as if they are "sticking up" for themselves. Even these high-strung babies will with time be able to calm themselves.

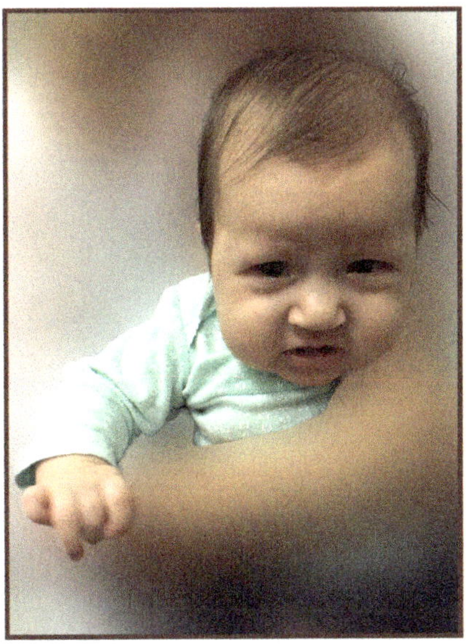

A mellow cry

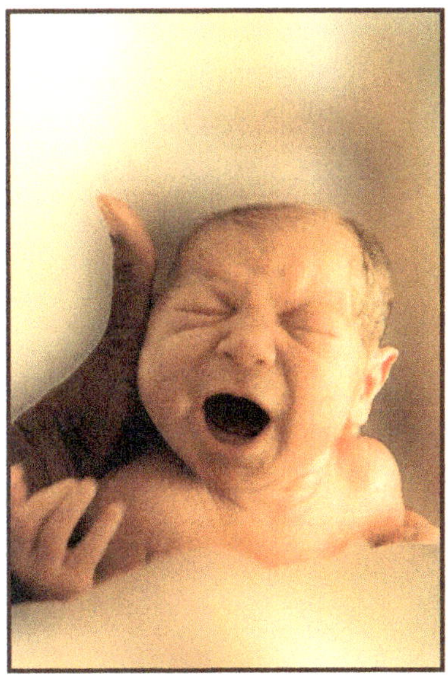

A high-strung's cry

Beauty exists in all temperaments. The high-strung infant may not initially take well to change; he may be very frustration-intolerant. Yet he can learn flexibility as he becomes older. What is initially an inability to tolerate change can, as an adult, become tenaciousness that benefits him at work or in other environments. With nurturing, his frustration intolerance can, for example, translate into good supervisory skills in adulthood.

Adjustment to Temperament

A Two-to-Three-Decades' Process

*"**What!?**"* you say.

Yep! That's it...a two-to-three-decades' process.

So, hold on for the ride!

And take a big, deep breath.

Initially, especially in the newborn period, it is the parents who must adapt. We must be there for them. Even later, we must remain flexible and tolerant, especially if we have been presented with a high-strung infant. However, with time, children with all types of temperaments must eventually learn to adjust themselves to live in the world of others. That's called "growing up." They must master their own temperament and use it to its best advantage to become socially acceptable to others so as to achieve, thrive, and flourish. That adjustment process can last at least for two, and sometimes (perhaps more likely) three, decades! The young adult's brain continues to develop into its mid-twenties.

Parents thus must help each child differently. For example, if a mother is on a stroll with two four-year olds, one high-strung and the other mellow, the high-strung child may run way out in front, forcing the mother to cry out, "*Wait, I can't keep up with you!*" The mellow one, on the other hand, may be dawdling along, way behind her, observing every little dandelion and blade of grass along the way. The mother finds herself shouting back, "*Hurry up, we'll never get there!*"

Certain aspects of temperament and disposition remain constant throughout life, such as adaptability or the ability or inability to accept and manage change, sensitivity and threshold to pain, tolerance for and expression of frustration, and intensity of activity and expression. While certain of these attributes may sound negative, they are not. Great strength occurs in being intolerant of poor performance when one is in a managerial position.

Delightful color comes in exuding one's feelings; as an adult, they can make, for example, an impressive speaker. These are powerful temperaments and, if they adjust well within their surroundings, their power can be quite expressive and creative. The mellow temperament as an adult can be quite calming, and organizing in difficult situations. **With parents' nurturing, all variations on temperament can flourish!**

Part III:
Other Actors in This Rite of Passage

The Anthropology

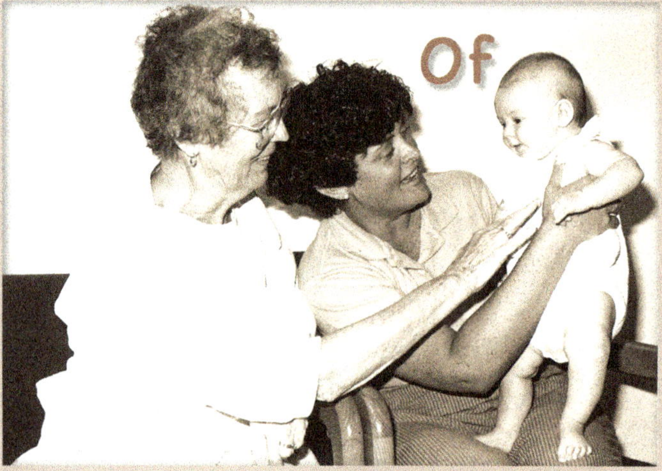

Of

the Mother's Mother

Chapter VIII: More Intrusion

Old Wives' Tales Abound

"If you let him stand like that his legs will bow and you'll have to have them broken and reset when he's fifteen."

"Push his ears back so they won't stick out."

"Rub olive oil into his scalp so his hair will become thick and wavy."

"Don't forget the 'evil eye!'"
(See "Evil Eye.")

When I hear these stories related as a new baby is brought in, I always ask, "*Which older relative told you this?*" Knowingly parents chuckle.

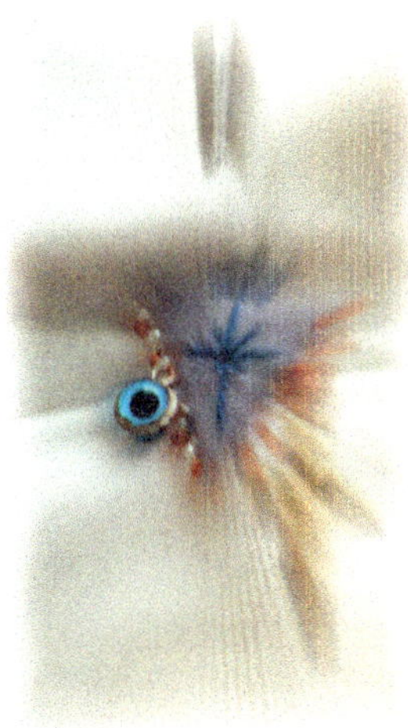

The Evil Eye

As a folksy part of all cultures' certain oral traditions known as "Old Wives' Tales" are passed down by the elders. Usually wise they are not; but almost always gifted with foreboding they are. As they say, it comes with the territory. It is part of the Rite of Passage. You must be hazed to join the ranks. You must be burdened with the same fears their grandparents and relatives traumatically taunted them with. It just goes on from one generation to another.

But parents, knowing these are experienced, trusted, and loving grandparents or older uncles or aunts, wonder still if the "tales" are true.

The question: Why do our elders persist in doing this?

Hypnotic Suggestions and the Wildest of Dreams

"Just after I delivered my first child, my mother came to visit. To support me she wanted to help out. I was looking forward to it. With great fanfare she arrived with presents. But it wasn't long before she began to offer me advice. 'Drink beer with every nursing, it helps with the let-down.' I hate beer. But I worried that if I didn't, I'd fail. 'Nurse her lying down or else you'll get big floppy breasts.' I really worried. She impressed me with how good she was at breast-feeding all of her children, and how late she had weaned me. I had felt fine before she began talking but the more she went on, the more I had this fantasy that I might actually fail. I wondered if it wasn't a challenge. She would also say, 'Don't get upset or your milk will dry up.'

"I'm an educated woman and I thought to myself: these comments feel almost like hypnotic suggestions. I wondered if she subconsciously was hoping I would fail. I wondered if those comments from my mother didn't come from envy that I could now have a child and she was beyond it and she resented me so much she let it out in these sorts of comments. I wondered if she were competing with me. I wondered if she wanted to be larger than life and perfect, someone I could never even hope to equal, not even in my wildest of dreams." (See also "*The Ultimate Loss Perceived,*" Success Neurosis, and the Anthropology of the Mother's Mother.)

I am sure that any given grandparent comporting as described above would be shockingly affronted if ever daringly confronted with the above mother's wondering interpretations of her own mother's behavior. But this is unbelievably seen time and time again. And one is left with the conclusion that those are fair interpretations of some mother's mother's behavior. (See the discussions around the anecdotes *The Carefree Socialite* and *The Ultimate Loss Perceived.*)

One imagines that it must be really hard for some grandparents to have the mothering role and to then have to relinquish it to let their own daughter grow thus allowing/supporting their daughter now in her new role as mother. The redefining of the mothering role into the grandmothering role—and the same is true for the fathering role—is often fought, or reluctantly accepted. It is always hard to change your own ego image of yourself.

Some grandmothers, and grandfathers, want to remain the hub of the wheel for the family. Some, even lovingly, will raise their children in a "rescue mode," as described in "Rescue versus Empathy," to the extent that their grown children will remain dependent upon them, even as they become parents (see *The Ultimate Loss Perceived*).

Very uncommonly a mother will raise a child to be impressed with his/her own illness, or limits, or little ability to stand on his/her own two feet without the mother. Then that child as a young adult and later as a parent remains dependent upon the now grandmother who has, to her satisfaction, now remained the powerful and important hub of the family. Furthermore, the reluctance of some grandparents to change from their old parenting role, can be a cause for competition with not only the new parents but also with their child's spouse and the spouse's parents.

Fortunately, most grandparents are supportive in a way where they offer help only when it is needed and advice only when it is asked for, thus allowing their children to be proud of their own ability to stand on their own two feet in this rite of passage. These grandparents are then proud of their children-now-parents' accomplishments. That is where they get their satisfaction as grandparents.

The Extended Family

Today's Family

While many families have close ties, some large, extended families can be too intrusive for new parents. Grandparents, uncles, aunts, cousins, and grown siblings may all live near, allowing them to celebrate cultural and religious holidays together, as well as this new arrival. The first pregnancy of a new couple preoccupies the parents' time and thoughts. And with delivery, in come all the congratulating, interested, involved, and advice-giving relatives. A young couple may suddenly realize the amount of time they have for their own life together has now become unbelievably brief. Thus, the infant may not be the only intruder into the new parents' life of intimacy. Also, if the couple has only had a few months together before becoming pregnant, the baby and the extended family may be particularly burdensome.

For others, the extended family may live farther away. The couple may then have the mixed blessing of being pleasantly isolated but without support, such as being there to help with childcare while you rest. Of course, if the relationships are good, these distant relatives may travel to be with the new parents and their child, but sometimes more often than desired. It's always a mixed bag, but hopefully there are more blessings than downsides.

Successful Grandparents

The Goal

Unlike the above story, many grandparents are often even better than they were as parents since their responsibility is limited to the times when the grandchildren are present. They've learned through their own parenting experiences. They often realize two things: 1) They are aware of their continued importance to their children; and 2) Sensing the touchy, vulnerable nature of new parents, they are wisely reluctant to express any unsolicited criticism or advice to their children in their new role. These grandparents, rather than being intrusive, are "in tune" with what their children need from them. They feel necessary in a new way. Thus, generations can hold onto each other and be mutually supportive.

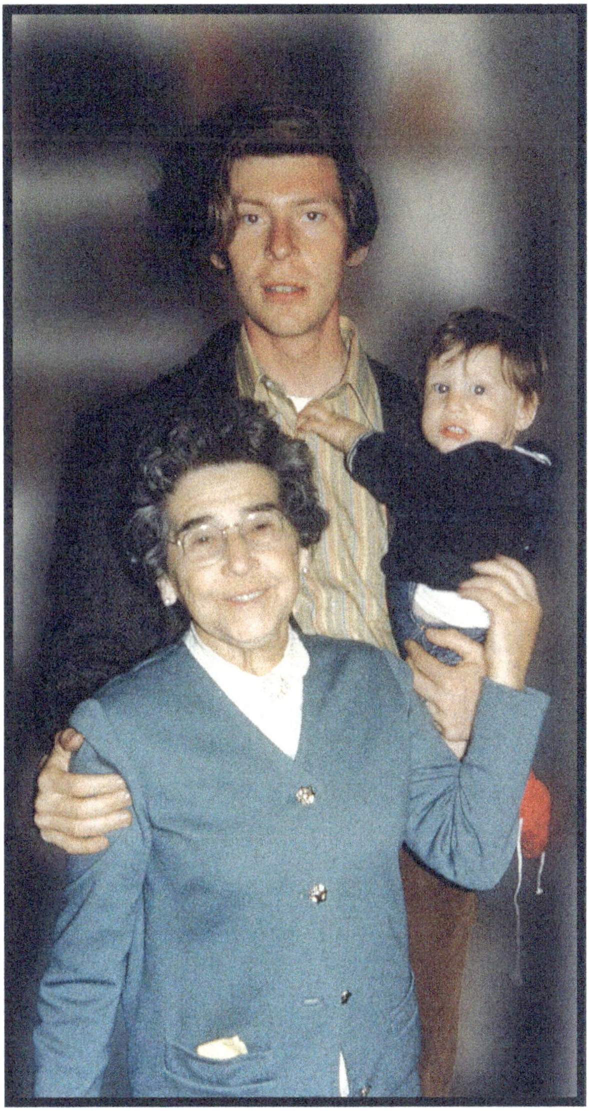

Yes. This is Mutual Support

Most grandparents are truly thrilled to become grandparents. It is a very special, proud feeling to see your own children go on to have children and to do well. These grandparents avail to help but do not intrude. They "shore us up," giving us only sought-after advice. They accept us as equals and serve as experienced, wise mentors when needed. They let us be autonomous and independent. They are not imposing. They teach by silent example. An example of helpful grandparents appears in the anecdote *The Ninth Month Vacation* (Book III).

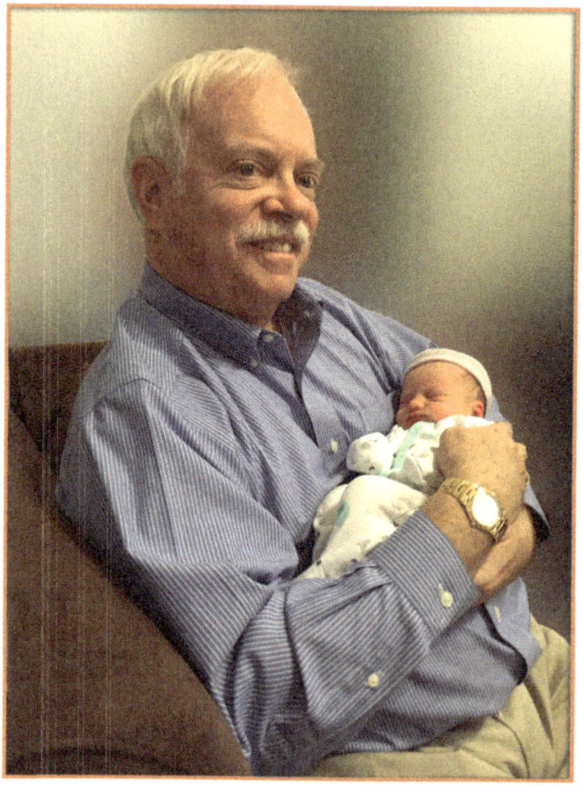

"This is hard to beat!"

The Obstacles

It is not easy to be a grandparent. These days, grown children are often educated away from home. Their training and jobs take them great distances from the nest, the village. They meet spouses who, often, may live in different cities. Some grandparents are increasingly disengaged from their children, moving to the Sun Belt and away from their children. All of these factors have contributed to a slight dissolution, in some instances, of the extended family.

On top of that there are more blended families, grandparents who have divorced and remarried and sometimes have new children with a different spouse. Nonetheless, the goal of the grandparent in this situation should be as a supportive, unobtrusive mentor.

The Internet world, however, allows many new parents to return, virtually, to their hometown, their village, while continuing to thrive financially. Generations can stay connected through various forms of social media, video chat, and email. They can again have the supportive advantage of grandparents, extended family, and friends. This is only helpful to a point, however, as demonstrated when the child is ill and grandparents who live at some distance away can't easily serve as immediate and 24/7 daycare back-up.

Giving Up an Old Role

While challenging, being a grandparent should mean augmenting one's role and not necessarily relinquishing being the parent of the new parents. The new role can focus on quiet empathy, so the new parents can make their own independent decisions without feeling regressed by "rescuing." (See the discussion around "*The Ultimate Loss Perceived*.") Grandparents can also be there for the grandchildren. They can still teach by quiet example without being intrusive. They can always be there when needed. They can always listen, without giving advice unless it is asked for. Sometimes they may feel that advice is truly needed; they learn to raise it as a question for the parent to answer. They are "in tune" with their children, now these new parents. But it can be hard, really quite hard to watch quietly as their children inevitably sometimes stubble and fall during this parenthood trek. And harder still not to say, "*I told you so*." But it is the parents' Right, in this Rite of Passage, to stand on their own two feet; and grandparents have to let them do that.

Grandparent Watching

Watching a grandparent in his or her new role is also an opportunity for the new parent to rediscover how a grandparent acted as a parent. While many are better grandparents than they were as parents, it is nonetheless an opportunity for insight into how one was brought up. The "ghosts in the nursery" can sometimes be spooked out as parents understand and feel the impact from the now present grandparents.

The In-Laws ... or Overcoming Soceraphobia

Needless to say, difficulties with inlaws have been there since the dawn of *homo sapiens.* A father's mother may be critical of her daughter-in-law's mothering. The mother's parents may be more possessive of their daughter and her child, and not mind the exclusion of the father's mother. And so on, and so on. But after having a child and feeling one's own investment in that child, most parents are bit more understanding of, and not as threatened by, some parents-in-laws' irritating reactions. These irritants may, hopefully, actually enhance parents' mutual support for each other and elicit a light-hearted sense of humor.

The Anthropology of the Mother's Mother

First, The Father's Mother

> ***The Father's Mother***
>
> *A grandmother had two sons, one of whom had married. This son and his wife had a little baby boy six months before. There was joy after the delivery, many celebrations, by all the relatives and friends. Life settled in, all was going well. The grandson thrived. The new mother talked daily to her own mother about all that was going on.*
>
> *The father's mother was, albeit cordially, slowly left out of the loop. The mother's mother came by daily to talk with her daughter and to play with her grandson. The father's mother was relegated to visiting only for two hours on Thursday afternoons. She became quickly and quietly sad and angry. She wanted a relationship with her grandson but felt cut out. Her*

> *son was back to work and presumably totally unaware of conflicts and, truth be known, did not want to be involved in family intrigues; nor did he want to deal with his own mother's anger.*
>
> *While the father's mother felt totally left out, the mother's mother was content and the mother was happy. The father's father listened to his wife's laments but, despite being furious about the way they were treated, felt he could do little.*

But after a bit of time it was brought into the open; and the issue was resolved...sort of.

Why "sort of?"

See what comes next.

Now the Mother's Mother

Anthropology studies of most cultures show the same pattern: The new mother always, assuming no pathology in the relationship, relates primarily to her own mother, if her mother is available. She feels she can safely share with her own mother who has known her since birth. She, knowing her own mother loves her usually unconditionally, can expose her own vulnerability issues and openly seek her advice. On the other hand, her husband's mother, being attached to her son, may not be always sympathetic to her daughter-in-law's issues. She may sometimes, in fact, be in competition with her. As one can see, this usual scenario does obviously tend to leave the father's mother somewhat out of the picture.

Being conscious of these issues may help to smooth the waters. It is all about "relationships and intrusions." Assuming reasonable relationships, an extended family can be supportive and not threatening. A mother, while appraising her own sense of security in her relationship with her partner and child, may evolve towards not being threatened and realize that grandparents on both sides can be very supportive when needed, both early on and down the road as the child grows up. So, if possible (and sometimes that is a big "if"), it may be wise for a new mother and father to keep up and be protective of relationships with both grandparents. The best question for making these decisions is: What's best for the kid, not only now but in the future?

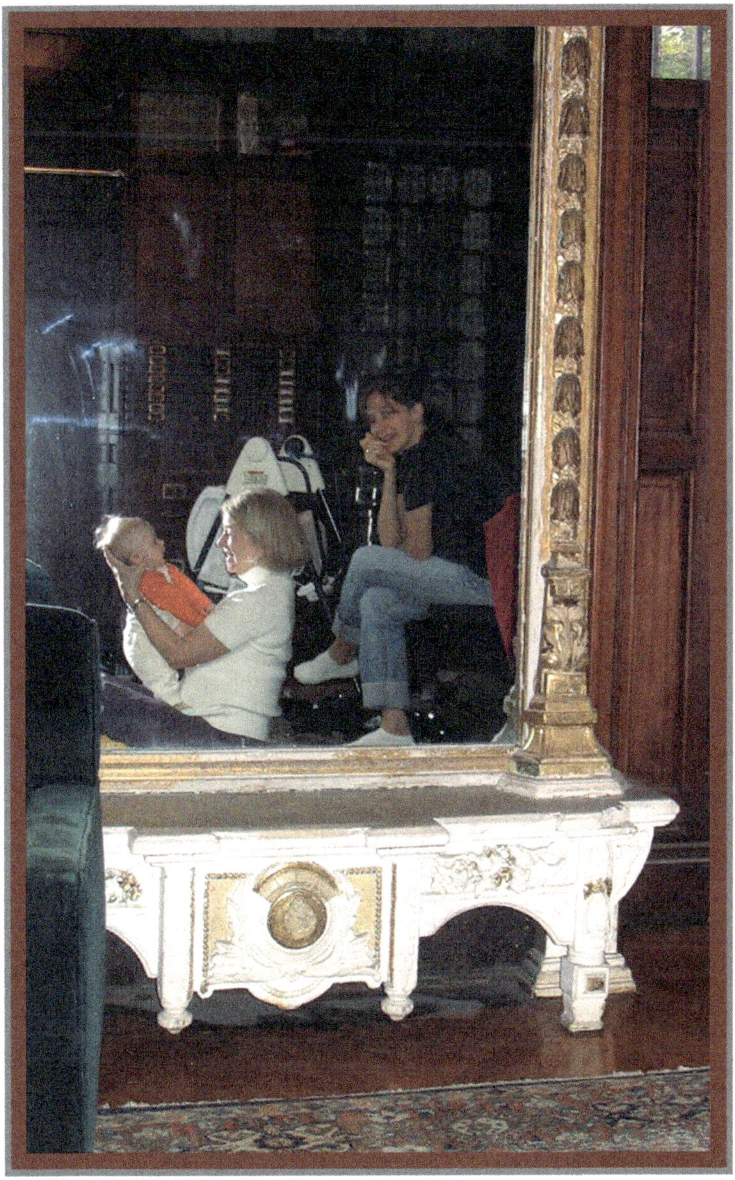

Question? **Do you think this is the mother's mother or the father's mother?**

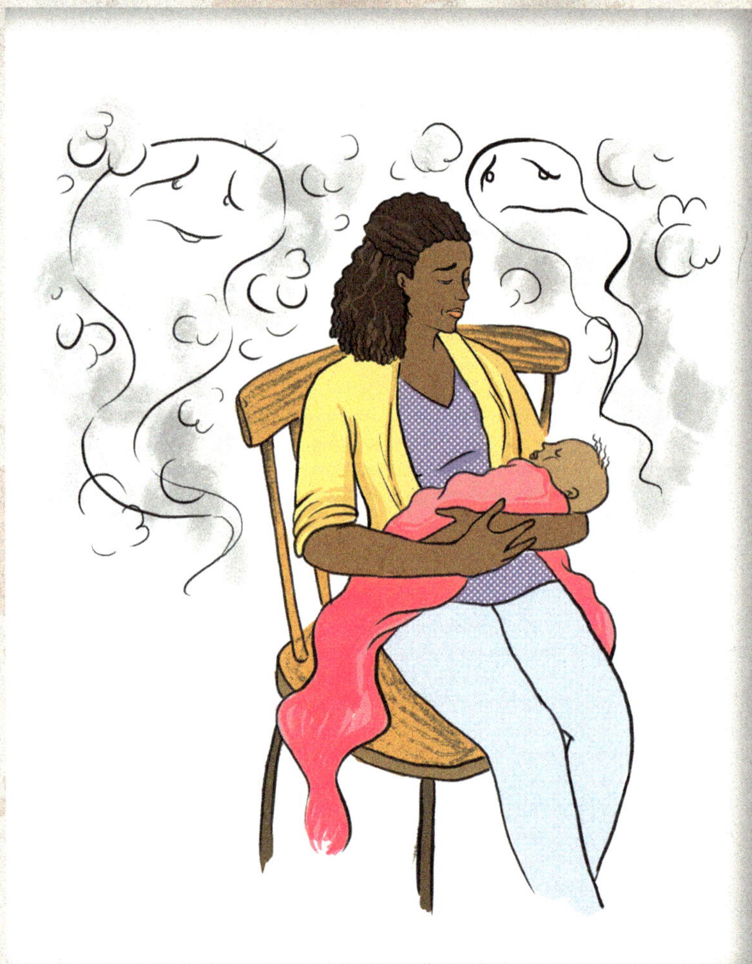

Chapter IX:
Ghosts in the Nursery

The Mother's Mother

The following story is one that we may not identify with at first glance. However, as it unfolds, it touches us ... regardless of our background or socioeconomic status.

> ***The Carefree Socialite***
>
> *Mrs. Fairchild was a smartly dressed, attractive young woman with the height and beauty of a model. She had been well cared for by her own family from the Deep South, and her affluent husband took over that role, assuring that none of her wishes went unfulfilled. She was extremely trusting and had done well with her life by following her parents' and now her husband's advice. She had no interest in working and even expressed scorn for it. She was quite content. Her favorite pastime was shopping. She was eager to have a baby; recently her friend had delivered.*
>
> *She became pregnant. Her life was happy. She was looking forward to having a perfect, warm, cuddly baby. She expressed being thrilled with the idea of taking her soon-to-be-born infant out shopping for the beautiful new baby clothing now available from France and Sweden.*

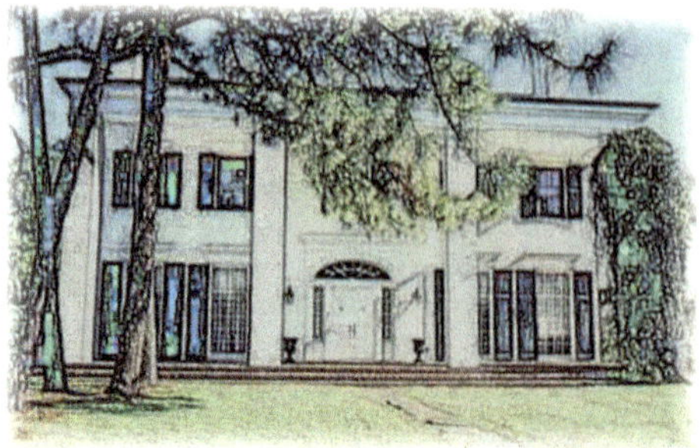

The Deep South

The delivery was tolerable. Her son, Francis, was beautiful and healthy. All went well for the three days in the hospital where she, as her friend had done, initiated breast-feeding.

Francis, however, developed problems after leaving the hospital. The first involved breast-feeding. It quickly became apparent that Francis had a high-strung temperament. His sensitivity to discomfort was obvious and disconcerting to him and his parents. He also had a moderately upsetting gastrocolic reflex (see glossary): After forty-five seconds of breast-feeding Francis would pull back and cry as if something terribly painful were occurring in his abdomen. Then, to everyone's distress, his sudden pulling away from the breast would initiate his Moro startle reflex (see glossary). Francis would scream desperately at his own lack of control over his newborn reflexes.

Mrs. Fairchild tensed with controlled panic because she felt as if Francis were rejecting her breast. Adding insult to injury, after Francis had pulled away and been somewhat consoled by burping techniques, he remained frantically hungry. Attempting to return to the breast, his cheek would hit his mother's arm, which set off his panicky rooting for a possible nipple on the close, warm surface of her arm. His head would bang up and down and from side to side against her arm. He would stiffen, arch backward, and cry inconsolably with a newly provoked startle reflex. This pattern would repeat itself, over and over again. Mrs. Fairchild was reduced to tears despite support and encouragement from her husband.

Mrs. Fairchild's mother came for a visit to help with Francis's care. What was a well-intentioned visit by grandmother turned into fiasco. Mrs. Fairchild's mother was scornfully non-supportive of breast-feeding. She found it distasteful. Her criticism was not limited to breast-feeding—she often reproached Mrs. Fairchild, expressing comments such as, "don't hold him that way, that's what causes colic!" ***Mrs. Fairchild later mentioned that her mother never allowed her to touch or hold her own younger brother when he was an infant.***

Mrs. Fairchild looked to her mother for support and instead received only scornful feedback. Mrs. Fairchild became even more apprehensive about breast-feeding and was especially reluctant to breast-feed in front of her mother. Her self-confidence became increasingly undermined. She was on her way to developing a very poor image of herself as a mother.

Francis's high-strung temperament evolved into burdensome colic at about three weeks of age. Mrs. Fairchild's mother had left, and Mrs. Fairchild sought advice from a range of sources. Her friends, who also enjoyed shopping and who were for the most part cared for by their husbands, were not endeared to child rearing. They told her, "Raising children only gets worse." Mrs. Fairchild was quickly becoming overwhelmed.

She was embarrassed to seek help from her pediatrician. For her, asking for help was admitting failure. Pretense was more important. She was mortified at having lost her composure, thinking she appeared incompetent as a mother. She shopped around for another pediatrician, only to return to her original one, even more embarrassed.

Mrs. Fairchild and her pediatrician worked together to uncover, dissect, and discuss her feelings. Although initially reluctant to relinquish her image of herself as a carefree socialite, Mrs. Fairchild was slowly able to show her distress and ask for her pediatrician's help. Through this process, she was able to develop more control, and appreciate Francis more.

Mrs. Fairchild and her husband were very attached to Francis. Mrs. Fairchild hurt when Francis hurt. When she learned that these were normal "symbiotic" feelings (see glossary), she felt less embarrassed and more human. She developed calming techniques for herself and for Francis. She learned about temperament differences and colic. As she mastered all of this, she gained self-confidence. She persisted and was able to successfully breast-feed. In time, she felt very positive about all aspects of her mothering.

She appeared sad at times as she became more self-confident and less dependent upon the not-so-good advice of her own mother. ***While she never talked about it specifically, she seemed to mourn the loss of the old dependent relationships that had been fostered throughout her own life.***

On top of all of these adjustments, she had to work through the loss of her very old dog, to which she had been dearly attached for many years. In addition, a wonderfully warm aunt who had been like a surrogate mother to her also died soon after Francis's birth. Managing the problems with Francis made her stronger, and she handled the other losses reluctantly, but well.

When Francis was around one-and-a-half years old she remarked, "Before, I enjoyed and always thought of myself as a 'socialite.' But recently a friend came to visit and said, 'Gosh, have you really matured.' You know, I really don't like being mature. I liked it the way it was. But I do feel good about it. I'm not sure I would have survived all of this without it. Also,

I feel like a better mother and Francis seems so much happier."

The Pediatrician asked her about her mother's last visit. She commented, "My mother is no longer critical of me, but she never praises me. But I know she is proud of me because she tells all of her friends and I eventually hear about it."

Spooking Them Out

On May 23, 1974, the famous author of *The Magic Years*, Selma Fraiberg, presented a historic paper. This paper, entitled "*A Ghost in the Nursery*" is considered landmark text for understanding the dynamics of how child abuse repeats itself from one generation to the next. The paper describes some very abnormal parent-infant relationships. It reaches the conclusion that "ghosts" were present in the nursery, affecting the behavior of the parents she was helping.

While Fraiberg's presentation illuminated the problems of severely impaired infant-parent relationships, it is clear to most child-care professionals that "ghosts" live in every nursery. Understanding, remembering, and discovering them in the mist helps to spook them out and enhance healthy parenting. In the anecdote, "*The Caribbean Connection*" (Book III), the mother had perhaps forcibly forgotten her experiences as a child. However, the feelings of those experiences lived within her as a "ghost" preventing her from reassuring her own son in his own separation fears. When she recalled her childhood experiences and compared them to her son's, she felt and relived them. Then, she was able to empathize with her son and separate herself from his feelings. Learning this lesson allows a new parent to hang on to the healthy models or aspects from their own parents and their own past. They can also gain from new, healthy models and new experiences and thus not repeat a possibly deleterious parenting pattern. This lesson is critical for parents who, in their own childhood, have been subjected to sexual, physical, or (far more commonly) psychological abuses (such as emotionally unavailable parents, for whatever reason). In the field these have now been given the collective acronym of ACE's, or Adverse Childhood Experiences.

The ghost(s) is most often the parent's own parent, usually of the same sex. Our own parents have an unknowingly potent influence on our self-esteem and our effectiveness in the parenting role. Their behavior as parents toward us, both when we were little and now while we are parents, in turn, influences how we behave with our own infants. Their approval and support, or lack of support, profoundly impacts how we feel in our own parenting experiences.

The story of Mrs. Fairchild is shared to detail the importance and influence of a parent's parent and the occasional occurrence of a grandparent's sabotage.

Mrs. Fairchild's mother found fault with her daughter's problems rather than being understanding and supportive. She castigated her daughter in her newly acquired mothering role. Indeed, she had not even been supportive during childhood (recall Mrs. Fairchild was forbidden to hold her younger brother). Mrs. Fairchild was raised as if incompetent, always needing her mother or later her husband; she was always taken care of and remained dependent as such. Mrs. Fairchild's mother was critical of her daughter's breast-feeding, appearing jealous of her daughter for succeeding at something she herself had not done.

This grandparent sabotage phenomenon exists. One can speculate that, for some grandparents, seeing their own children successfully parent may be a threat to their image of themselves as parents. (See Chapter IV and the *"Ultimate Loss Perception,"* and Chapter VIII for "Old Wives' Tales.") Perhaps some grandparents may be insecure feeling no longer needed nor powerful. If they are no longer needed they may, feeling useless, fear further separation from their children. Perhaps grandparents, too, have ghosts in their nursery that are reawakened with their child's childbearing, or that their own anxieties as young parents are coming back to them. Or they may simply feel that they are the only ones who can do it; their way is the only right way. It seems as if it might be *"all about me [them]."*

Other aspects of this story are important and will be discussed elsewhere. For example, the "Wish versus Reality" phenomenon is seen when Mrs. Fairchild longed for a cuddly baby and instead received a high-strung, colicky infant. Mrs. Fairchild evolved from a highly dependent role to achieve independence. Growing from a leftover-from-childhood stance into adulthood, she felt joy and accomplishment mixed with sadness and loss for what she gave up to become a very good mother. She had to make up time and give up on being dependent on her mother and husband in order to see her son happy.

Most grandparents are supportive, loving, and not imposing. Others treat us as they did when we were little. Others compete with us; maybe that competition began actually when we were born: The Intruder Complex for them. Something to ponder.

A Distant Ghost

Mrs. Weiner planned to return to Norway, her homeland. She was taking both her one-year-old daughter Annika and her three-year-old daughter Beata to visit both sets of grandparents.

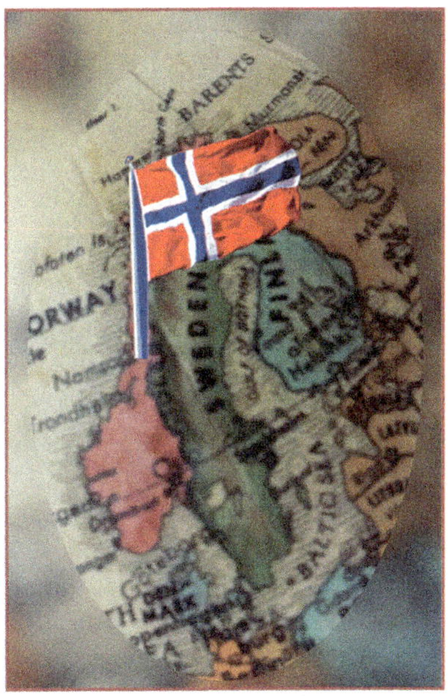

The Ghost in Norway

Mrs. Weiner was looking forward to the trip with mixed emotions. She was elated to be returning to her homeland. Yet, while she was happy to be able to visit her in-laws, she dreaded visiting her own mother. She softly lamented, "Doctor, I'm thirty-eight years old but I feel like I'm reduced to a child when I'm around my mother. She is so unsupportive of my breast-feeding and so critical of me in general! I want her to love me and respect me, but I don't feel she does. It is very much on my mind, even here far away from her."

Such feelings can be a powerful presence, a ghost, ever present in a new parent's mind. Part of Mrs. Weiner did not want to grow older. To mature would be to lose her mother (see "The Ultimate Loss Perceived"). Mrs. Weiner wondered aloud if she wasn't raising her daughters to remain dependent on her, just as she felt she was with her mother.

She went on the visit, returning later to report that, despite her fears, it went surprisingly well. She was able to separate herself from her mother, who astonishingly then respected that independence.

Mrs. Weiner understood her mother felt a continued need to remain a mother. She felt ridiculous, experiencing the feeling of being a child herself even though she was thirty-eight years old. Yet she was powerless, even at a distance, to control these feelings until she experienced her own feelings with her own daughters. Mrs. Weiner was not previously able to separate herself from her own mother until she saw and felt the separation and independence conflicts her own children were having with her. Upon returning to Norway, contrary to her fear, Mrs. Weiner did not lose her mother but actually gained her mother's respect.

The Father's Father

Wheezy, Part II (Continued from Book I): Wheezy's Grandfather

Before Wheezy was born, her parents had affluent aspirations. Mr. and Mrs. Wishfergeld were both employed and shared the conscious aspiration of attaining a financially successful life together. Jolted were their well-orchestrated ambitions when Mrs. Wishfergeld discovered she was four months pregnant, despite taking birth control pills.

Both parents were depressed...and furious. Mr. Wishfergeld wanted an abortion. His wife disagreed, crying, "Don't you want my baby?" She could not pursue the abortion. Wheezy was born.

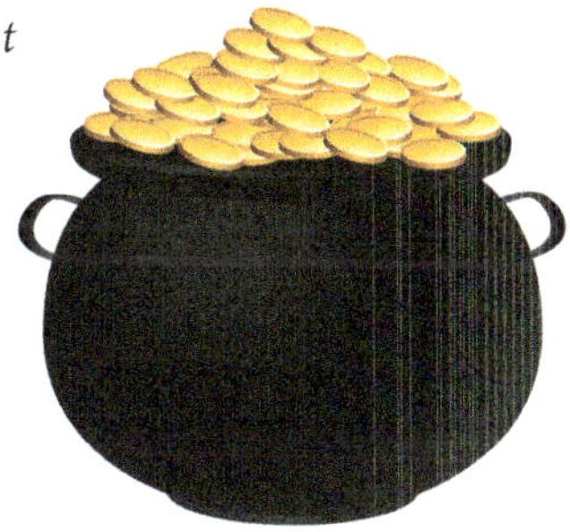

In the first weeks, Wheezy received a lot of attention from mom. The father was warm and attentive but jealous that his wife's affection was directed toward his breast-fed daughter. He felt completely left out and retaliated with pouting possessiveness. He had not wanted this infant in the first place, and now he was disturbed that the infant was here and breast-feeding.

By the time Wheezy was six weeks of age, both Mr. and Mrs. Wishfergeld were back to earning money. But, at seven weeks of age, Wheezy developed severe recurrent asthma, which required repeated hospitalizations. While she had initially been breast-fed, wheezing began when her diet was occasionally supplemented with a soybean formula. (Wheezy, while not diagnosed as yet, had developed a severe legume allergy to the soy.) Her medical problems intensified her parents' mixed feelings of love and resentment by requiring them to spend large amounts of time away from their work to care for Wheezy.

Both parents experienced feelings of guilt. Mr. Wishfergeld felt awful for not wanting Wheezy and for being furious with her for demanding so much time because of her illness. Mrs. Wishfergeld felt responsible because Wheezy may have inherited the allergy and asthma from her; and, also, she was the one who insisted upon keeping the pregnancy. Secondly, the wheezing appeared to be exacerbated by Mrs. Wishfergeld's smoking. Mrs. Wishfergeld felt frustrated and wanted her daughter to be well. Yet, she could not stop smoking. Compounding the problem, Mrs. Wishfergeld did not follow the pediatrician's advice to feed Wheezy a more expensive but non-allergic formula, which contributed to the difficult task of arriving at the correct diagnosis.

Wheezy's mother wished things were better and was angry when they were not. She panicked and was unable to cope whenever Wheezy became sick. Wheezy's arrival had intruded upon plans for financial success and now Wheezy's illness was yet another intrusion.

Mrs. Wishfergeld's tolerance level dropped as she became more and more depressed. She overreacted with fury to small deviations in Wheezy's asthma. She felt trapped, and her anger would often find a nearby target in the doctor. Desperate for quick relief, Wheezy's parents shopped around for different doctors.

Wheezy's father, while initially jealous during the early healthy weeks, became empathetic and supportive as Wheezy started wheezing. He spent a lot of time at home or at the doctor's office so his wife would not be bothered. He helped with the housework and changed diapers. He nurtured Wheezy and helped her through her illness while trying to offer emotional support to his wife.

At the same time, he felt sabotaged by his own father who would deride him for changing diapers or cleaning up the kitchen: "That's women's work. Why's a man like you doing a thing like that?"

Mr. Wishfergeld became less tolerant, not only of Wheezy but also of her demanding illness. Feeling no support from anywhere, he became punitive. The parents became angry at each other as no resolution appeared in sight.

Wheezy thrived despite her difficulties. She grew despite her allergies. Her parents became refreshingly open. They were able to work out their emotional problems with the help of their pediatrician. As the story evolved, the legume allergy was detected, and treating that problem solved her wheezing. Mrs. Wishfergeld had the same allergy and is also no longer wheezing now that she herself has eliminated legumes and smoking. Wheezy is now a delightfully impish, pretty, and bright five-year-old girl.

Wheezy's story highlights Mr. Wishfergeld's journey of growth. He possessed a remarkably strong wish to handle his daughter's illness, enabling his wife to keep working and attain their common aspirations. For a time, he endured his own father's [the ghost's] criticism and lack of support. But his own father's faultfinding made Mr. Wishfergeld depressed and resulted in punitive, displaced anger in the form of verbal attacks on his wife and infant. Only after seeing what was happening could Wheezy's father gain control of these feelings. Only after spooking out the ghost of his own father could he be happy and proud of his parenting, and of his protective bonding to his daughter.

You

are

Guilty...

of

Guilt

Chapter X: Guilt and "Guilting"

Guilt Is Now a Verb

Wheezy's parents felt guilty that they resented Wheezy's conception. They felt guilty about being angry that Wheezy's birth and illness had intruded into their financial aspirations. Wheezy's mother felt guilty that she may have caused Wheezy's asthma. She was at times furious and blamed ("guilted") her pediatrician for not solving the problem. She guilted her husband at times. He, in turn, was furious and blamed her and Wheezy. Wheezy's father's father guilted Wheezy's father for doing a woman's work and chided him for not acting like a man.

How does all this guilt and blame come about? We all "guilt" ourselves and others (so much so that I now use guilt more so as a verb and not a noun!). Guilt is an almost universally felt response to unusual, difficult, uncontrollable situations. For example, the parents whose child may have developed pneumonia may ask, "If I had insisted that he wear the sweater underneath his winter jacket, wouldn't that have prevented the pneumonia?" An older sibling of a patient with a malady may ask, guiltily, "Was it the last time I hit him that made him sick?"

It is quite difficult for all of us to accept that some of life's problems, while we wish and strive to control them, are beyond our reach.

Now that is a difficult concept to accept! We forget that, for example, pneumonia is not a problem that can be assigned to weather or clothing. And, of course, no one intentionally causes pneumonia. We are not that powerful! It is as if we wish we were that powerful, so that we could have prevented it from happening. And since we could not prevent it, we now feel guilty, wishing and, more importantly, assuming that we were that powerful... since we should have been that powerful.

Guilting Others

Besides guilting ourselves, we also guilt others. Grandparents often make us feel guilty when they themselves are the ones who feel guilty. They may portray both jealousy and guilt. They may feel disappointed that, as parents, they did not do things as well as the current generation. Like Wheezy's grandfather, they may feel that they should have prepared us better. But to save face, to avoid making a mistake in front of one's own child, they may rather want to guilt us so that it appears to be our fault, our problem—not theirs. Guilting others is thus a way of dealing with helplessness—a feeble attempt at undoing what has happened. It is a way to protect the vulnerability of one's sense of self. Thus, guilt and guilting results from a feeling of helplessness, a fear, and a failure to have done what we think we should have been able to do.

We see guilting constantly in the field of medicine, particularly in anxiety-producing situations. For example, if something goes wrong in the delivery of a baby, the pediatrician may tend to blame the obstetrician. The obstetrician may accuse the pediatrician, and the parents may want to blame one, the other, both, or themselves. The physicians may even want to blame the parents. It is far easier to presume someone else's negligence rather than to accept the normal human mishaps of life. And it is difficult to accept that no one can be absolutely perfect and in control all the time. We thus fault ourselves, or others, as if we should have been able to protect ourselves from a bad outcome.

The psychological term is "projection," but for the sake of a common understanding of this phenomenon, I call it *guilting*. The "guilter" is, in fact, feeling guilty but projects it toward someone else, to "the guiltee." By guilting someone else, it is then not the guilter's own fault.

Guilt and guilting exist in all ordinary families. Parents do this to each other; friends and grandparents can do this to new parents. Most of the time it is harmless, even amusing. But sometimes it can hurt first-time parents who are still fragile in their new role.

Sadness, depression, and even anger can follow guilt. Parents are often concerned that their not-always-perfectly-loving feelings will impact, possibly irrevocably, the psychological development of their baby. A parent may then feel guilty not only for having those feelings but also for the harm they think the feelings may cause the infant. Thus, a parent can become even more sad and depressed. For some of us, if simple sadness or acknowledging fear is not a permissible feeling, we may become angry and blame someone else. Thus, a mother may become angry with the father, doctors, nurses...or her infant, even blaming the baby as described above in the "Homunculus Phenomenon."

Guilt feelings are also commonly evoked from parents' competing desires. A mother, after delivery, may feel left with a shapeless body not at all to her liking. She desires the best for her infant, but also has a wish to live up to her image of herself. However, the continued need for adequate maternal nutrition, essential for breast-feeding, may prevent her from regaining the physical image she had of herself prior to pregnancy. A conflict emerges and the mother may suddenly resent her own self-sacrificing even though she wants the very best for her infant. Guilt may then punish her, as if she has "selfish" concerns. **Thoughts for solutions to come!**

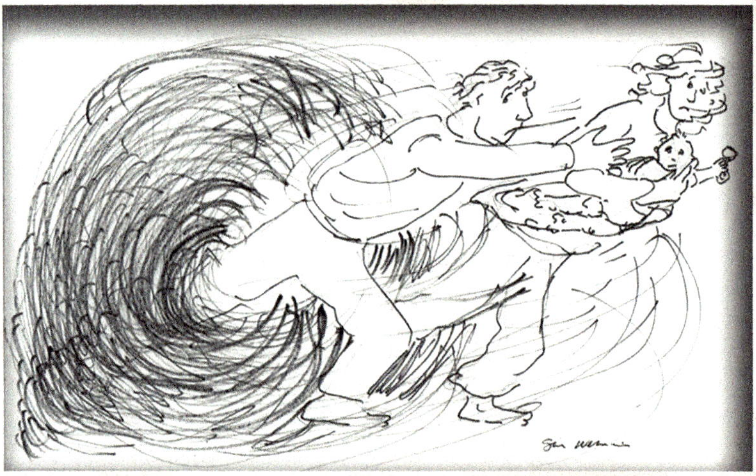

Part IV:
Out of the Fog

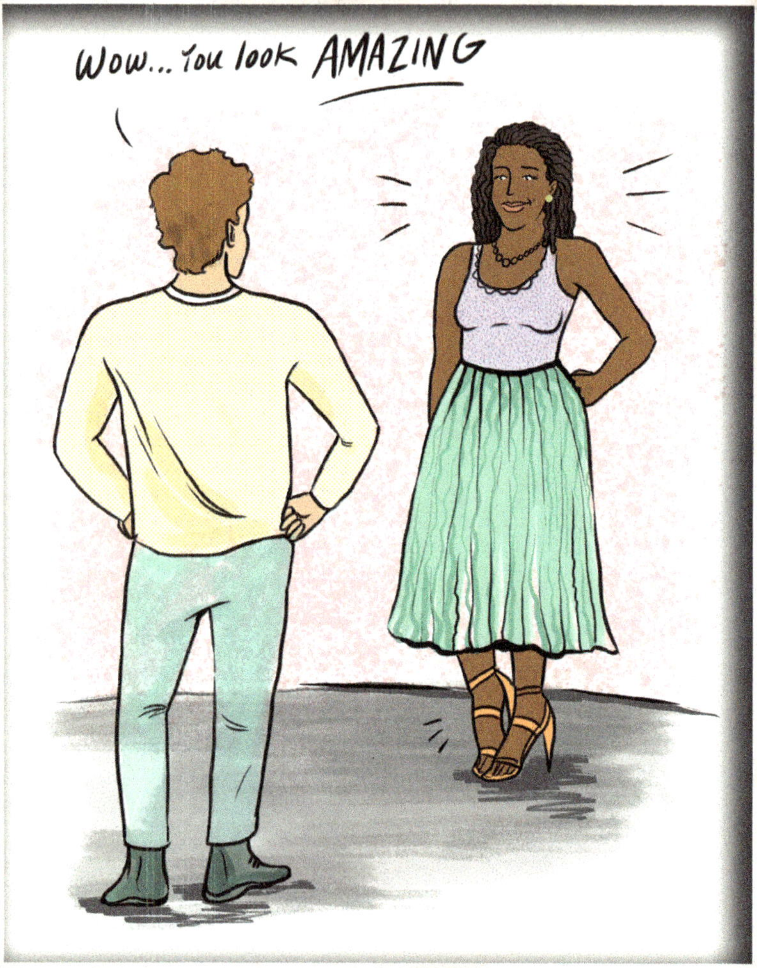
WOW... YOU LOOK AMAZING

Chapter XI: Strengthening Yourself

Surviving the Intruder Complex

Talk About It

The Intruder Complex can blindside you; it is most often unspoken or unconscious. If parents can recognize these feelings, a better chance of mastering them exists. Otherwise, these feelings can manipulate and wreak havoc on the new parents' life of intimacy.

When the Intruder Complex leads to feelings of jealousy and/or a diminished intimacy, it is healthy to (1) talk and simply share feelings and (2) to spend some time alone together. Sometimes, partners feel they should be strong enough to handle all of these feelings alone. Fathers/partners may believe it is a sign of weakness or a lack of adult maturity to express, "*I need to talk with you...I would like to spend some time together, with just you...I could use a hug!*" Those feelings are important and worth considering. It takes maturity and courage to verbalize them. If it is hard to talk, write letters to the other.

A new mother may feel that her husband/partner is a grown adult who does not need her as much as the infant does. Of course, both parents need to support each other. But sometimes all is sacrificed for the mother-infant relationship. **It's as if the child is put upon an altar**. The driving force for this is love for the child. But another driving force could be to perform perfectly in this rite of passage in becoming a mother, so that we look good to all others (See the anecdote *"Trying to Please Everybody, but not Harry."*). A mother may, in aspiring for perfection, forget and unconsciously abrogate her role as a partner. She may want to avoid Breast Feelings and sex and closeness with her partner as she falls in love with her new infant. But is that healthy for the family, including for the child who will perhaps thrive best in an intact family? Love is always other as well as self-regard.

In the mother/mother/child family where one is birth mother and the other in the role of spouse, these feelings can be intensified. The non-birth mother may, being in the father role, feel "odd-man-out." But layered on top of that may be jealousy that she is not, or could not be, the actual birth mother when in fact she is also a woman. Clearly, in protecting the relationship, it is best to take this issue up openly in planning a child. The spouse in the m/m relationship did not donate sperm. Unfortunately, sometimes in anger the birth mother may then claim this child as just hers (See Narcissistic Rejection in Book I and in the Glossary). Prior planning for a timely legal adoption avoids a lot of contention (Laws vary per state; and lawyers specializing in this are available). Anticipate, and share the feelings lovingly!

Spend Time Together

This need not be a major production. It doesn't need to be expensive; it doesn't even necessitate a great deal of time. It can mean sitting for fifteen minutes alone together on the back porch, lunch out together on a Saturday, or a brief walk together in the afternoon. Parents can be exclusively breastfeeding and still get out for a brief time between feedings.

An understandable reluctance exists in planning any alone time. Your free hours and minutes are already so limited. Moreover, a mother may be reluctant to use a babysitter feeling (or being told that), "*no one else can care for this baby like I can.*" That is true: But you are only using a babysitter for a very limited amount of time; you are not putting your child up for adoption. So, only a few minutes or a few hours here and there can be helpful. "Overprotective" parents not using a babysitter need to ask themselves not only why but who are they protecting, themselves or their child; and what are the consequences if this "over-protectiveness" continues? Will their child grow up fearful or with a good sense of security? If a father or partner's work schedule makes it difficult to find time, make an appointment. When someone else attempts to intrude on this scheduled private time together, parents can then say, as they would in the office, "Sorry, I already have an engagement at that time. Let's find a better time."

Now to sex

Discuss it **out loud, or actually write it down and send a letter to each other.** What will you do and when will you do it? It's even better, if you have a chance, to discuss this before delivery. Make sure each parent's needs/wants are at least addressed. And then, what can you both do to accommodate each other? What if you can't be physically intimate in your "usual" ways for a while? What will you do as an alternative? What if one can and the other can't? What can be done as a loving compromise? There are thoughtful, loving ways to handle this. What if there is no libido? (See "Loss of Libido," below). But even that loss can be shared. What if a postpartum depression causes a loss of positive emotions as well as a loss of libido? Even that can be shared thoughtfully. Neither partner needs to be alone in this journey.

It is not selfish to maintain, or even enhance, your life of intimacy together. A strong, close relationship between parents can be enjoyed and is indisputably healthy for the infant's current and future happiness. One mother noted, *"There's probably a lot to be said about modeling a healthy relationship with your partner for your child. I imagine we all want our kids to grow up with healthy expectations about how to interact with a partner (including romance and respect)."*

Compliments, Gratitude, and Compassion

How difficult is it to share compliments or express gratitude or demonstrate compassion? Consider the impact of these statements, which are often forgotten (or at least not expressed out loud):

"Wow, you're doing an amazing job."

"You look great."

"Thanks for what you do."

"Thanks for that hug."

"Thanks for the help."

"You know, what you're doing has got to be tough."

It sure feels good and supportive when you hear it, or *say* it for that matter. How often do we forget the power of these ideas when entrapped in our own thoughts?

Empathy for happiness is wonderfully supportive. Most often empathy is given when support is needed to do something difficult that needs encouragement. But it can be really nice when it is also given honestly and supportively to your partner who has accomplished something that is simply expected.

> ***"Oohs and Aaahs"***
> *My husband needs to merely hold our daughter in public or push her in a shopping cart at Target and he gets warm smiles and "oohs and aaahs" from admiring mothers. They think he is performing a wonderful act of fathering and caring for our sweet girl. That is NOT the case when I am out with her, as it is merely expected of me.*

Society presents us with different expectations to live up to (or fail at). Yes, it is nice for a mother to acknowledge and engage/support her partner in his triumphant parade through the aisles of Target. But is he also understanding societal pressures and expectations, and supporting his partner? Maybe she needs a hug or a pat on the back, too. Or better yet to empathize with her happiness with her own simply expected accomplishments: *"You must be really happy with how well you are handling all of this. It's really great!* ***You*** *must be really proud of yourself! Well, I am proud of you!"*

In addition, avoid righteous criticism. The other parent is doing their best and will probably do no harm; and maybe their approach has merit. So, in that case, silent support and a silent hug may be the wisest. Resist statements like, *"Let me do that, I know how to do it."* Such statements are subtle put-downs. No one wants to feel incompetent.

All of this is major! This is critical for teamwork. This is what you do for each other in team sports. Right? This is what you do in business collaboration, or any joint endeavor, if you want to be successful. Right? So why not do it in the parenting endeavor.

The Paternal Instinct: From Possessor to Protector

For the father/partner, the newborn becomes real with birth—a living, breathing person who actually exists in the world. Initially, a proud-of-a-miraculous-accomplishment feeling engulfs partners, followed by close physical contact. Almost every partner experiences that deep, strong thrill when the infant quietly snuggles safely and securely on his or her chest. It is a special feeling to watch him fall asleep there, contentedly, with his little head to one side, his knees drawn up, and his tiny clenched fists held closely to his body. You can actually feel the Biochemistry of Love and Bonding, the "rush." Also, a feeling of strength and increased closeness comes over a partner when he or she can successfully calm their infant.

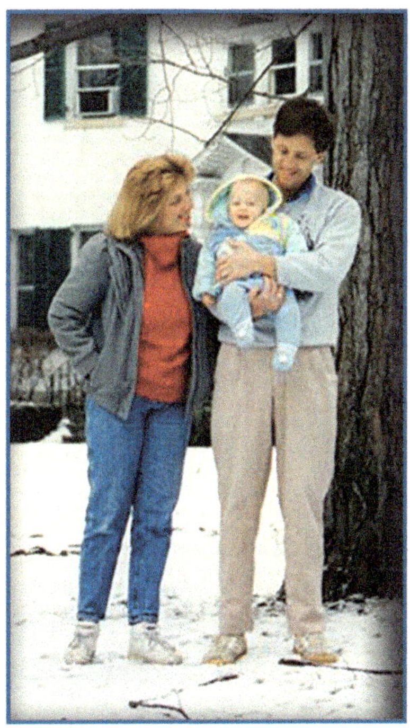

Now the Protector

Thus, resolution to The Intruder Complex also comes with the partner's strong attachment to the new infant. It evolves when the partner incorporates the growing reality of the infant into his or her own sense of self. The partner becomes possessive and protective of the new infant, also a result of the biochemistry of bonding. The partner emerges strong. Many express, *"It is really strange. For the first time, I can understand how someone, myself included, could actually kill to protect the mother of their child and the child if they were threatened with harm."*

This quietly formed bond can become jarringly apparent to a partner. The mother may want to take their new infant to visit out-of-town relatives. The spouse/partner may not be able to leave his job; and, while initially looking forward to time alone, he may find himself missing them terribly. The partner left at home may even become depressed and angry, which can affect his everyday actions and interactions at work and with friends.

Postpartum Depression

> ***Damn***
>
> *"Damn. I felt a little miserable after the first little guy came along. But, damn, I feel miserable with this second little guy. I don't know what to do or say or how to behave. My husband is wonderful and supportive but I just feel awful and cry all the time. I worry what my older kid thinks. I sure am not available to him, and I can barely feed this new one. I have no reason to be depressed, but I am really low. I don't want to take medications because I am breast-feeding. I feel alone; I don't know what to do."*

There are degrees of postpartum depression. It may not exist, it may be simple ("the baby blues"), it may be hormonal, or it may be complex.

Not infrequently a mother may initially feel, *"I don't love this kid...how can I love this kid? He's like a little alien."* But with a bit of time, and the first smile and cuddling, the parent is snared in the process of bonding.

More often the hormones are tough. The withdrawal of the pregnancy hormones occurs after delivery and is often like menopause or PMS (premenstrual syndrome). Moody weepiness can engulf the mother. Impulsive, rabid anger/hostility is not uncommon. Usually just talking about this with your spouse, the doctor, the doula, or relatives or friends can help. It often disappears after a few weeks or so; but sometimes oral 50 mg of daily OTC B_6 along with 12.5 mg. of hydrochlorothiazide can be extremely helpful (consult your doctor).

Postpartum depression may, however, become complex. Emotional baggage from a mother's past can be forced to the surface with the birth of a child, and must be confronted. Egregious examples include the physical or sexual abuse of the mother as a child or teenager. Having a newborn sometimes then evokes all sorts of posttraumatic stress disorder–like (PTSD) conflicts between a mother's repressed conflicts and protecting or neglecting her newborn. Or it can be the issues of "Success Neurosis" and/or *"The Ultimate Loss Perceived."* Such issues usually require some professional help.

A parent's depression has a face associated with it. A depressed parent cannot be as emotionally available. So, an older sibling of the newborn may perceive, upon looking into his parent's face or feeling the parent's lack of joy, the depression as anger and rejection. That can be addressed by explaining to that child that it is not his fault. It is just that mommy is sad from some of the changes, or from feeling sick, or from something other than the older sibling. Let him know it is not his fault, that he is not the cause of it.

Loss of Libido

> *"I have two children, a two-year-old and a four-year-old; and since the birth of the first one I have lost all interest in sex. Why is that and what do I do?"*

Loss of libido in women is not infrequent, is often not spoken about, not always "shared," and is not easily solved. It is not a simple plumbing problem like erectile dysfunction, which can frequently be quickly mastered with medications. It is usually multifaceted, complex, and not uncomplicated. No single "love potion" seems to be out there.

Sexual arousal for women is often "responsive," rather than due to anticipation, yearning, or horniness. So, sexual arousal may not happen until being actually involved in the sexual activity; in other words, the arousal and stimulation after the activity is initiated then leads to desire. So, while initially uninterested, the arousal can come after getting involved in sex.

Also, variations in frequency occur with couples. Sometimes it's frequent and sometimes infrequent; and individual couples may be comfortable/ happy with either. The problem comes when one partner wants more and the other is disinterested and the lack of desire remains so even after attempts to arouse.

Sexual interest and arousal varies with age. But other factors can be operating, such as emotions from interpersonal relationships, exhaustion, job stress, low hormones such as low testosterone even in women (in women testosterone is important for yearning and getting horny), and medical problems. Even certain medications are notorious for the decreased libido (for example, SSRI antidepressants and some birth control pills). Emotional problems, such as preexisting constitutional depression or reactive depression like that seen from the losses described in the anecdotes "*Finally*" and "*Career Mother,*" can clearly influence libido. Issues as described in Breast Feelings and Success Neurosis, or other issues such as the doomed desire for perfection, and even PTSD brought to the surface by childbirth may operate. Multiple causes can coexist and may require sorting out. Excessive alcohol intake, alcoholism, and drug addiction are obvious major contributors.

Sex therapy has been shown to help. Changing medications or dosages may be required. Addressing underlying medical or emotional conditions may be helpful. Vaginal estrogen creams and lubricants can help with vaginal dryness. As you can see, for women this is not simply a plumbing problem. So, to sort out the situation, professional help by someone experienced in this area is, more often than not, needed.

Breast Feeding: A Few Tips Not in Most Books

Avoiding Sore, Cracked Nipples

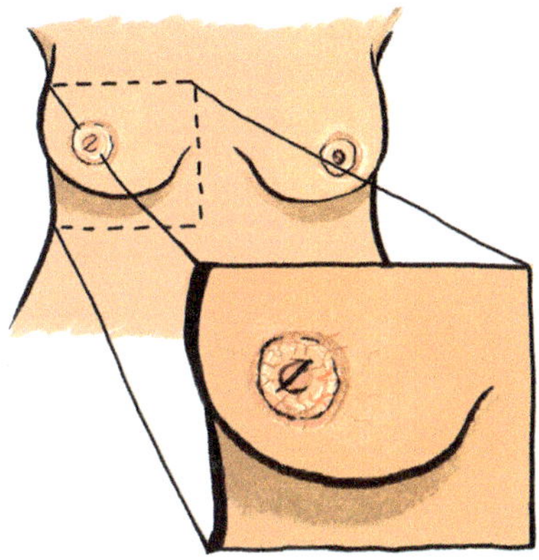

Notice the diagonal crack in the nipple aligned with the infant's suck if initially held perpetually in just the cradle or cross-cradle position.

Book I and Chapter V of this book cover initiating breast-feeding, and particularly breast-feeding the high-strung infant. But then what happens? *"When will he sleep?" "I have heard that he can get his days and nights mixed up." "What do I do?" "Can I prevent problems?"*

You may ask in the hospital, *"How long do I leave him on?"* Some will answer, *"As long as he wants."* Sounds nice. But soon after arriving home you may experience sore cracked nipples; and this whole wonderful experience is no longer joyful and pleasurable. To avoid this problem, try to remember, and that is not so easy, to dutifully rotate through the three feeding positions. That rotation evenly distributes the pressure points of his sucking lips around the areola. If you only hold him in the same cradle or cross-cradle position and allow him to suck forever you may quickly have a bleeding painful crack diagonally on the nipple where it was perpetually squeezed between his upper and lower lips/gums (See the graphic depiction of this).

Also remember that "frequent brief feedings are better than long infrequent ones." Look again at the graph on breast milk production. You don't need to do more than 6–10 minutes maximum per side. Any longer than that may contribute to sore nipples. Besides that, by going longer he is not getting any more milk. But all of this becomes better as your nipples adapt by three weeks or so. See the in-depth discussion of this in Chapter V.

Refusing One Side?

Sometimes there's a reason; and sometimes not. But some newborns will only like one breast and resist the other. It may be an inverted nipple. Regardless the reason, and usually there is not, insist on his starting on the resisted side. It can be unhealthy for you if he takes only one side and not the other; it can result in issues like clogged ducts and mastitis on the unemptied side. So, insist that he take at least 2 minutes on that reluctantly accepted side before going to the other; and always, always start on that side. If he starts on the easy side, he'll want only that side. So as not to worry, see the graph (Chapter V) and note how much breast milk comes out in the first few minutes.

Do not give up on insisting on the reluctant side first; and then let him stay there a bit longer (ever increasing seconds) each time before letting him have the easy side. He will eventually adapt. On the other side, the easy side, stop after around 8 minutes. If he wants more, insist that he go back to the first side. This will work; but you should always insist on the reluctant side first; and start that insistence the minute you notice this problem. If, after the feeding, you are still engorged on the first side, you can pump it to empty it. Save and freeze the pumped breast milk for when needed at some future time. If you can, before starting to breast-feed, also pump the reluctant side for just a bit of time to relieve any engorgement, it will facilitate his latching on.

If while resisting the first side he conks out, pucker your lips and repeatedly blow **very forcefully** with your breath straight into his face. (Don't worry about germs; within 24 hours of birth he already has every germ you have.) This causes him to wake up blinking with a slight inhale, and becoming sufficiently awake to attempt latching on again. Your partner can also drip either water, formula, or pumped breast milk just above and onto the nipple as he is attempting a latch. It will whet his appetite and entice him to initiate latching on and sucking.

Falling Asleep on the First Side?

Now this is a very good problem. It means you have a great milk flow. So much so that he falls asleep full, from the first side, and is uninterested in going further. So, what do you do? As mentioned, it can be unhealthy for you to have an unemptied breast. So, start with just giving two minutes on one side **by the clock**, then immediately switch to the other side. But stop after 6–8 minutes on the second side; and, if he wants more, go back to the first side. At the next feeding, start on the opposite side. After a few weeks, your breasts will adapt and he will only need the usual 6–8 minutes per side. Don't go beyond 10 minutes on either side; he's hardly getting anything after that (see the figure on the Milk Ejection Reflex in Chapter V of this book).

Going to Sleep with Rocking, Walking, and/or Feeding?

While this is an often-preferred way to get the infant to sleep, you can buy problems doing it. The best way to instill "good sleep habits" is to do it from the start and have him learn how to go to sleep from the awake state without motion or being fed or held... but not alone without your being there.

The problem often is that you can get into chasing your tail: Let's say he falls asleep only by being held and fed. But then as you put him down in the crib to continue his sleeping, he is, of course, only in the light-phase of sleep and thus will reawaken with a startle reflex as he feels himself hitting the mattress. Erg! Then you keep repeating this back and forth until he falls asleep now with total exhaustion. Or you have to, as some do, drive him around in the car or put him on a vibrating drying machine (both options take place in his car seat of course) for a far longer time until he is finally in a much deeper phase of sleep where putting him in his crib will now not arouse him.

All of this usually does not make for happy parents. So, it is best to try to never even start with these habits. Just swaddle him very tightly using two blankets (see Book I for methods) and put him down and talk soothingly to him. Or sing, or turn on some music, or simply let it be quiet but with your soothing, empathetic, and soft voice occasionally in the background.

He will, within a short time, learn and adapt. He will then, having mastered that, actually be happier in the long run.

You can do the quick fix now and pay the price later. Or you can do the prevention now. But if you do get into this habit, don't worry. It can be worked out later; it just takes a bit more energy if done down the road (a topic for Book III).

How Much Breast Milk Is He Getting?

In Pediatric Medicine, we have some complicated mathematical formulas to figure out how many calories and/or fluids babies need. We use these calculations in the hospital when giving intravenous fluids, for example. But I have pulled all of those together for you. Below is a clear, understandable calculation for determining how much breast milk a baby is getting, assuming he is growing well.

The simplified version by Peebles:

Just take his weight (from the last office visit) in pounds and multiply it by 2.5. That will give you a rough approximation of the intake in ounces needed per 24 hours to reach the weight he is at.

2.5 times weight in pounds

=

number of ounces needed per 24 hours

Why is this helpful? Well, let's say you want to go out with your partner for lunch and you have pumped breast milk. Then you can tell the babysitter just how much to offer him from the bottle while you are gone. Or let's say you have gone back to work and are breast-feeding but supplementing with some formula or pumped and stored breast milk; this tells you how much to leave with the day care people. So, let's say he is feeding 8 times per 24 hours; simply divide the calculated amount per 24 hours by 8 feedings to get the number of ounces needed per individual feeding.

Here is an example:

> At you last doctor's appointment let's say he was 12 pounds. Multiply that by 2.5 and you get 30 ounces per 24 hours. If at that point he is feeding only six times per 24 hours, then simply divide the 30 ounces by 6 feedings. You then would offer 5 ounces of breast milk or formula in the bottle for that one feeding, or perhaps top it off with 6 ounces, just to be safe.

Or, let's say you have become worried about his growth and have supplemented with formula and think, even though he is growing well, that you are hardly putting out any breast milk since you can't see it or measure it unless pumped and then given. Just do the calculation. You then subtract the amount of formula given per 24 hours and you have the obligatory amount of breast milk you are actually putting into him for him to be at the weight he is, assuming he is growing along the growth chart available from your pediatrician. That may indeed relieve your worry/anxiety.

> Using the example above of a twelve-pound infant, that means he must be taking in 30 ounces (12 x 2.5) per 24 hours to be at the weight he is. If you are only giving, say, 3 supplemental feedings of 4 ounces per feeding, then you are giving him 12 ounces of formula (3 feedings of 4 ounces each) per 24 hours. You calculated that his total need for 24 hours is 30 ounces; and you are giving him only 12 ounces of formula. That means he is actually receiving 18 ounces of breast milk (30 – 12 = 18 ounces) from you even though you can't see it going in. He should, must, be receiving that much to acquire his current weight.

Or, let's say you're completely breast-feeding but curious as to how much you are putting out. Just do the calculation. You will be astonished! By the way, this simplified calculation using the factor of 2.5 only works for the first four or so months of age, but it is reasonably good for these purposes.

Burping

"How do I know if he has burped, or needs further burping?"

Now for a bit more fun: Some years ago, a pediatrician wrote a serious, albeit to me humorous, note about this published in the prestigious *New England Journal of Medicine,* of all places. His favorite two methods were eliciting (1) Tympany over Traube's space or (2), my favorite, the Succussion Splash.

Traube's space is in the upper left quarter of the baby's abdomen, named after/by Ludwig Traube (1818–1876). Tympany is like the sound of a drum when tapped with the tip of the middle or fourth finger. Try it; it's easy to do. Take your middle or fourth finger and get used to tapping that area. Then tap the knee, or another part of the abdomen. Notice the dull sound on the knee and the drum sound over the Traube's-space part of the abdomen if an air bubble is present in the baby's stomach before he has burped. That drum sound becomes duller after the burp when the air under the drum is gone.

Now for the Succussion Splash. Pick your baby up under the arms while also holding his chest. Then hold his abdomen close to your ear. Then gently shake him, like you would a bottle with some liquid in it, to hear if you can hear the milk in his stomach slosh about because air is still in his stomach. If the air is gone after burping, you will not hear the slosh sound.

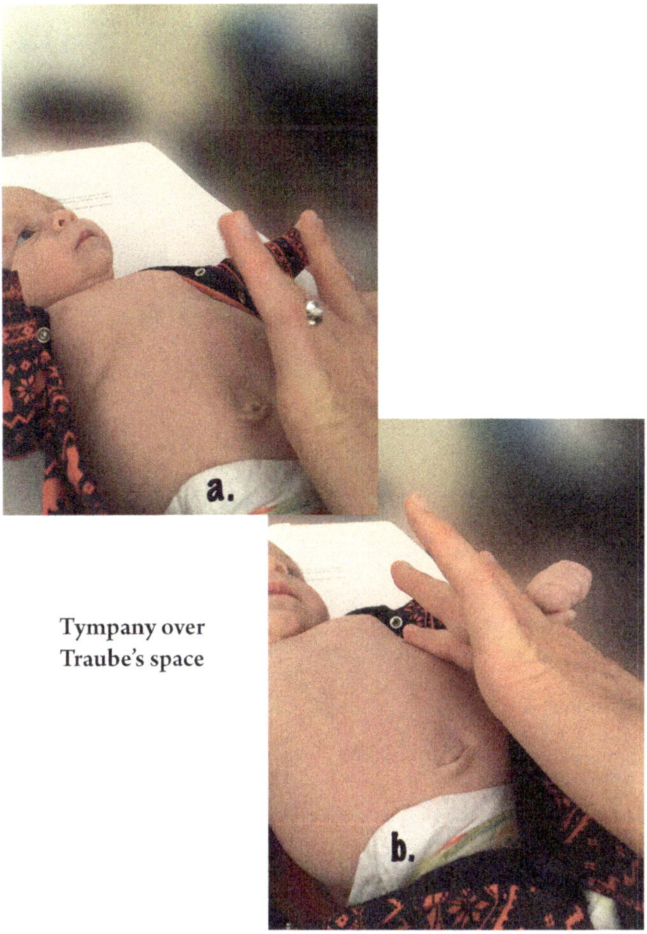

Tympany over Traube's space

All that aside, if he is hiccupping, he has burped and you missed it. Seriously. Little infants don't always give you a "high school or college-type" burp. You must watch them very carefully to notice this but some burps are just puffs of air coming almost silently from puffed-open lips. When the burped air exits, the now milk-filled firm stomach comes up and bumps into the dome-shaped diaphragm muscle at the bottom of the chest. When that muscle is irritated hiccups begin. So, if he has hiccups he has burped; you missed it; and you don't need to attempt further burping. (See Book I for a nice way to hold him for successful burping in the seated position.)

"Can I Enhance His Sleeping Through the Night?"

"Yep!"

Aim for a combination of "demand" and "scheduled" feedings.

Well, what does that mean?

When you go to a breast-feeding class or when you read about breast-feeding, you will hear those terms. Scheduled-feeding means you would wake him up and feed on a fairly rigid schedule basis, such as every three hours by the clock. Demand feeding means you would simply wait until your newborn demands to be fed; and then you would feed him.

Here is a problem that can evolve with a first born, but sometimes even with a second or third child: As they start to consolidate sleep, they can evolve to sleeping during the day coupled with being up all night feeding. In other words, they have their days and nights mixed up! That's fine for them but you are up during the day as usual, but then you are also up all night feeding. That is not a sustainable scenario. That does not lend itself to a pleasant life. Ok, so what happens and how can that problem be avoided?

What happens is that at some point during the day they start to sleep for a just a bit longer interval between feedings. You say to yourself, *"Great! I can read and have a cup of coffee, or I can pay some more attention to the older one."* Sounds wonderful. But then they sleep more and more during the day and suddenly have the days and nights mixed up.

To avoid this and aim for a good night's sleep, different approaches are available. But what I have found most successful is the following: (Look at the figure with the Breast Feeding Schedule.) During the initial weeks starting around 6 a.m., feed by the clock every 2–3 hours (wake him up to do this) but only 6–10 minutes per side. Burp for five minutes; and then you are done with that feeding. Do this by the clock up until 11 p.m. at night. That part is "scheduled feeding." But after that 11 p.m. feeding, let your infant wake you up (That's "demand" feeding).

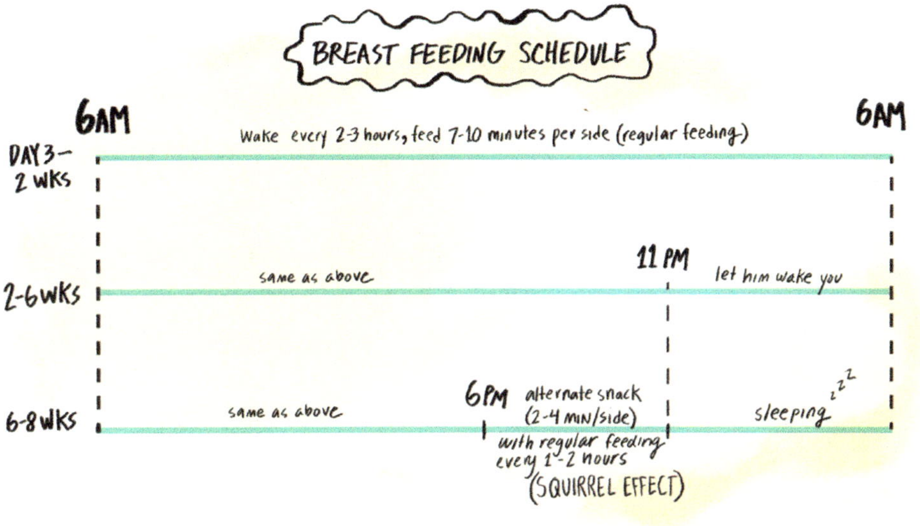

If you do this assiduously, what will happen is that he will slowly consolidate his sleeping into the nighttime. Gradually each night he will slowly extend the time of sleep from 11 p.m. to roughly 3 a.m., and then to 4 a.m. or so, until he is sleeping through from approximately 11 p.m. to around 6 a.m. That will happen around 2 to 4 months of age. It may happen sooner if he is more on the mellow side of temperament, or later if he is on the high-strung side of temperament.

This combination of day and evening "scheduled" feeding followed by nighttime "demand" feeding enhances his sleeping through the night and prevents his getting his days and nights mixed up. If during the day and evening time he wants to feed sooner, then simply give a 2–4 minute per side snack. Also, again see the milk production curve in Chapter V and notice that even a short snack will (1) stimulate a hormone pulse to produce more milk next time and (2) give him 50–80 percent of a regular breast-feeding. (See the figure on the Milk Ejection Reflex in Chapter V)

But, and there is always a "but," you will initially have to pay a price for his sleeping through the night. I call it the "squirrel effect." It is as if he were a squirrel storing away nuts for the wintertime. As he achieves sleeping through the night, the common pattern for him, from 6 p.m. to 11 p.m., is to want to feed every hour or so. It is as if he needs to squirrel away the milk so he can sleep through the night after the 11 p.m. feeding. Well, that could drive you crazy, or make you think something is really wrong with him. That's also when your partner comes home and wants to sit down and relax with you. But alas, the house is crazy with this ravenous infant.

Also, occasionally around six or so weeks of life there is an infant that may initially start with the "squirrel effect" without yet sleeping through the night. And you are wondering, *"What is going on?"* But that pattern is sometimes the prelude for sleeping through the night. So just be a bit patient for a few days. If worried at all for some reason or still worried after a few days of waiting, obviously discuss what's going on with your health care professional.

"But this 'squirrel effect' is driving us crazy!"

There is a way out that still gives you time to yourselves in the evening.

"Tell me, tell me now!"

Well you know how milk is produced. (See the figure on Milk Ejection Reflex in Chapter V) So the answer is straightforward: Simply alternate between regular feedings of 6–8 minutes per side, and 2–4 minutes-per-side snacks as you feed him through the evening.

So...if at 6 p.m. you give him a 6–10 minutes-per-side regular feeding but then he wants to feed again at 7:15 p.m., then give him a simple snack of 2–4 minutes per side with 5 minutes of burping and put him down to rest. That should only take a total of 15 minutes. So you can then go back and relax for a bit. But then at, let's say, 8:30 p.m. he wants to feed again. Then give him that regular feeding of 6–10 minutes per side. So you flip-flop through the evening between regular feedings and snacks up until about 11 p.m. or so; and then he will begin thereafter to sleep at night.

Don't forget he also grows in spurts. So at times either during the day or evening, he will want to feed extra. If that happens and it is before an expected feeding, first try the "airplane" calming technique (see Book I for pictures and an explanation, and see the glossary). If that fails to stall him until the next scheduled feeding, then simply give a snack as described above. Then stick to the regularly scheduled daytime and evening feedings. Not only does that give him a significant amount of breast milk but it also stimulates more milk production for the future, which will then take care of his needs for and after that little growth spurt.

Solving Breast Feelings

The Goal, Not the Process

All mothers and fathers want happiness and good health for their new infant. That means nurturing the newborn and taking care of all his needs because he is unable to survive without help, and he is unable to survive happily without solace for his irritations. The goal of breast-feeding is to satisfy the new infant's nutritional needs. What also comes with this nurturing is the critical warmth, the holding, and the closeness involved in the bonding process. That warmth and closeness can also be achieved with formula feeding. So "bottle propping" with letting the infant feed himself by himself while not holding him is not at all encouraged.

Breast-feeding should definitely be encouraged. It offers (1) the perfect nutrients for body and brain development, (2) the antibodies that suppress viruses (especially intestinal viruses), and (3) the warm closeness of the infant to the skin of the maternal breast.

That being said, others must respect mothers who opt not to or cannot breastfeed, or who choose to mix breast-feeding with formula feeding. More often than not, very good reasons exist for those decisions. The elucidations of many of these reasons are laced throughout this book (and also are in Book I). If formula feeding is chosen and, if that results in happiness, attachment, and health, the ultimate goal has been achieved. (See *"Everybody's Entitled to My Opinion,"* and related stories and discussion in Chapter III)

Another phenomenon that can occur with pregnancy is the perception by some mothers that the infant, as if an alien, has possessed her: *"He has taken over my body."* Breast-feeding can reignite the feeling of the alien takeover after delivery: *"I don't want to breast-feed at all. Enough is enough."*

Some mothers must be on bed rest to prevent a premature delivery, in some cases for months. Others may have incredible nausea and vomiting from prolonged and intractable morning sickness. The pregnancy has become anything but sublime. Understandably, a mother may then want her body "back to herself." Thus, feeling the need for a break, along with a desire to finally enjoy this infant, she may opt to not breast-feed. These decisions must be respected; they are important for bonding.

Further Solutions

Share problems with your partner. **Talk.**

Dripping, even squirting, breast milk during sexual intimacy can be disturbing to both the mother and the father. Perhaps it might be best to incorporate it into a novel, non-guilt-ridden sexual fantasy. Some fathers even express the desire to suck on the engorged breast as part of sexual play. This may be abhorrent to or enjoyed by the mother, or considered only the infant's territory. But, if dripping or squirting is upsetting, either nursing or pumping immediately before intercourse can easily empty the breasts and avoid the problem.

After delivery, the first sex with her partner may be an anxious moment for mothers because of a mixture of feelings. Some women may have less vaginal secretion after delivery, both because of these feelings and the lower estrogen levels that follow delivery. A lubricant, or even saliva, when used on the labia and in the vagina, may make intercourse less painful and more pleasant. (See *"Finally!"* in Chapter I.)

Warm, intimate, caring emotions are linked to sexual feelings within the mind and body. This is true for men and women. All the above feelings are frequent and real. There is nothing to be ashamed of or feel guilty about. Creative, non-harmful sexual fantasies are common, perhaps universal. There is no reason to feel guilty about fantasies. Feeling guilty about sexual fantasies is a residual from childhood that, hopefully, we are able to be more accepting of as adults. Select fantasies can often be shared and enjoyed between willing partners.

Talk. Talk. And talk again. Understand your feelings and those of your partner. See the section above on Breast Feelings. Understand the impact of "nipple territory." Learn to understand the significance of the Grading System, and the fallout evolving from this Rite of Passage and the Intruder Complex. Reading and understanding the anecdote *The Ultimate Loss Perceived* can help.

Above all, talk and talk and talk with your spouse. Share your feelings while respecting each other's, regardless of content. Don't always offer advice or solutions—often times just listening and sharing is all that is necessary. Learn to give and take. *"Love is other and self-regard,"* as the philosopher Thomas Aquinas thoughtfully stated.

It is always best for parents to talk together and share feelings even when it is difficult, even if one feels rejected, displaced, or misunderstood. The wish is that the unpacking of these feelings will lead to more successful breast-feeding.

Working Outside of the House?

Good News and Bad News!

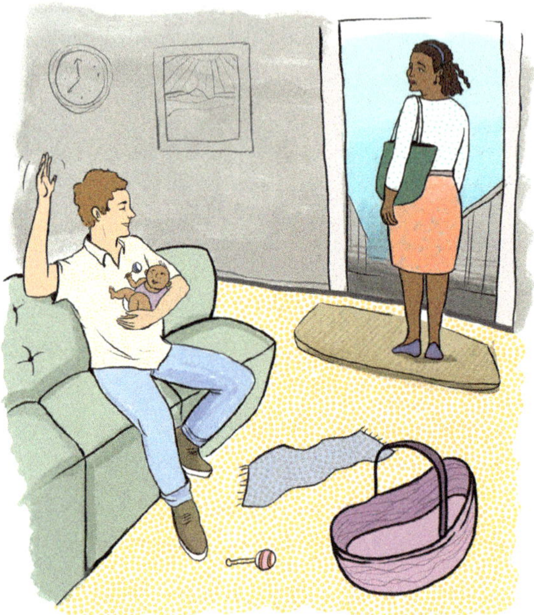

Not always easy!

First: The Good News

A new era has emerged, with many choices and lots of flexibility. Young women, more than ever before, agree that they are looking at a myriad of options that simply weren't there before. Parents can have a baby and still work. Employers offer infant-friendly return for work. Some even make it possible to have the baby at work. Better parental leave is acceptable and available, often for both mother and father. More and better paying jobs are available to new mothers. Many mothers also can afford to opt to stay home. Lots of options for daycare are available. Young fathers have a far more egalitarian outlook to childcare. So now almost everything is acceptable, and can be worked out. And with older siblings, in a way it is easier; you have previously gone through the process of reaching and implementing decisions on parenting.

Next: The Conflicts

The problem is in the choosing. The problem is that it may be impossible "to have it all." Usually way before delivery the waffling over these issues is somewhat resolved. Obviously, most opt to stay home for "maturity leave." But then there is that decision of whether to be a stay-at-home mother versus returning to the work force in the adult world. Some feel relief with staying at home; some feel relief upon going back to work. Some feel they can and want to remain home with this new bundle. Others, while loving the new bundle, want to or need to rejoin and exist in, for at least part of the day, the world of only "grown-ups." And there is always some sadness and worry. Also, while there is always some guilt, there is usually less nowadays: people can enjoy their jobs and feel they are no less a mom or dad.

The good news also is that many people now respect either decision, while before some in one group might have demeaned the other group (for example, working moms look down on stay-at-home moms and vice versa). People understand and can empathize with most everyone's feelings, realizing that whatever a new mother decides, it is not reached without some conflict or worry (see the anecdote "*Career Mother*" and the discussion around the "crisis of change"). Now with the above being a wished-for ideal world, one mother with lots of experience in both working within and outside of the home disagreed:

> ***"I Don't Think This Is True"***
>
> *"... by the way. I think there is a lot of judgment between these groups. 'I don't know how you can stand to be a stay-at-home mom. I would get so bored.' Or, 'I don't know how you can work knowing someone else is raising your child. I could never do it.' The judgments are usually pretty passive-aggressive, or disguised within backhanded 'compliments' or 'humble-brags.'"*

Again, competition and the Grading System! Erg! Not helpful for anyone, not even for the one feeling the need to justify their own position by being critical of others. A total waist of energy that can be redirected in a more wonderful supportive direction. It's hard enough without this.

Remember what was stated at the beginning of this book:

We are all parents. And we all have our children in common.

Those going to work must surmount some preoccupying, formidable, and worry-burdened barriers and the details involving the logistics of two working parents: Arranging childcare? Making list upon list of what is needed and when? Developing contingencies for when the child is sick? What is the division of household and childcare efforts, such as who's getting the groceries and how do we coordinate our schedules? How do we communicate and work, do we use texting and even a common iCalendar?

And then there is hardly a mom who does not feel at least some guilt about going to work away from her/his child. Usually the first times are really sad and somewhat difficult. Joy is there in being at work. But the real joy comes with reunion when everyone, usually, is excited to see you upon return home. And you are excited to see baby upon return. That's kind of special! But as one mother astutely painted the reality:

> ***"It's a Mixed Bag."***
> *"If you drop your kid off at daycare and they cry when you leave, you feel really guilty about "abandoning" them there. But if they are not at all sad to see you go you feel sad* **(and/or perhaps angry)** *that you've been so easily replaced and forgotten. Same for the end of the day: When you pick up your kid from daycare and they don't want to leave (a sign they had a great time), you're sad because they didn't miss you. But if they are rabidly eager to go home with you, there can be lingering guilt about having left them... Ugh."*

An old Swedish saying applies to the above conundrum. The English translation: *"No matter which way you turn, your backside is behind you."*

If a mother stays at home she worries she will not have it all: She will miss competing and wonder what is going on in the adult world of her previous employment. She will miss her old friends at work. She will be left behind.

Her husband can then sometimes become her only link to that world. He comes home and, while seeking the solace of being home with his wife and child, may upon walking through the door be barraged with questions about what **he** did at work. However, now there are blogs and Internet groups and local groups that often help fill that gap. But the stay-at-home mom nonetheless is entering and adapting to a new playground. She is home with the baby, there not to miss anything that happens in his development.

But no matter what options are chosen, change is tough, especially depending on your own temperament. As the mother above said, *"It's a mixed bag."*

But More Good News

Very important: no decisions are immutable. They need not be permanent. **You can change your mind.** You can be flexible. You can think about things and decide to decide later, or try one approach and then another. For example, do I want to be part-time or full-time, one day a week, 2 days? All decisions do not need to be made right away. You can try something, see if it works, and then change if it's not working.

How Do I Handle Feedings?

Sometimes it is just plain hard. You should figure out what you want and what to do to get there. But then there are the feelings. Erg! The first issue that requires resolution is daycare: Who's going to take your place caring for the baby, and possibly an older child as well, when you are gone during the day? Are you going to transfer to formula feeding, come to day care to breast-feed, or send pumped breast milk to be given by bottle? But then you have to get that all organized. There is the pump: what kind, and how does it work? Where and when do I pump while I am at work? What will it do to my supply? All that will need to be sorted out. (BTW, some pumps are covered on some health insurance plans. So, check out your benefits.)

Later on, you may want the flexibility, whether you are going back to work or not, of using a bottle with either formula or breast milk. That requires planning. Infants, particularly those tending toward a high-strung temperament, will refuse the nipple of the bottle and scream forever to return to the breast if they were breast-fed exclusively for more than two months or so.

So how does one manage that?

If you want that flexibility, then it is wise to establish breast-feeding by exclusively doing it for the first three weeks or so to make sure all is going well. **Then** introduce the bottle with either breast milk or formula and use it once a day, and definitely **no less** than once every other day even if, at that point, you don't actually need the flexibility.

If you go beyond using the nipple of a bottle at least every other day, or you introduce the bottle late (after two months or so), it may not work. This requires effort. Some will feel it is just easy and more enjoyable to continue breast-feeding. But there is a different suck required for the nipple of a bottle than the suck necessary for the breast. If infants have even a smidgen of the high-strung temperament, they get set in their ways very early on and do not like change. If you want them to be adaptable later on, you should introduce the variation early and get them used to it. They must *stay* used to it so you can implement it later, when you really do need the flexibility of offering either pumped breast milk or formula from a bottle.

It is possible to introduce solid foods and some cup feedings as early as three months of age along with continued breast-feeding, if you have not introduced the bottle early and they refuse the bottle. Talk to your pediatrician about how to do this. You can then breast-feed in the early morning before work and again a few more times in the evening after returning home from work. For fluids during the day, you can give them by a sippy cup or a small plastic medicine cup. Think about not feeding after late night. Everyone needs sleep; you do especially if you have a new child and are back to work as well.

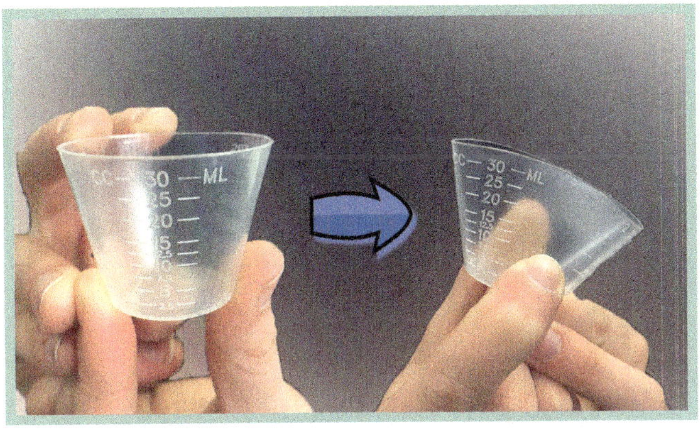

Squeezable small plastic medicine cups now used for feeding to avoid "nipple confusion"

Then there are the feelings. All of this can drive you a bit crazy. It's best to think about it and plan, ahead of time. But not to worry, some solution is always available, even if the planning went awry. As mentioned above, should you need to, you can introduce solid foods a bit early if your exclusively breast-fed two-to-three-month-old adamantly refuses the nipple of the bottle.

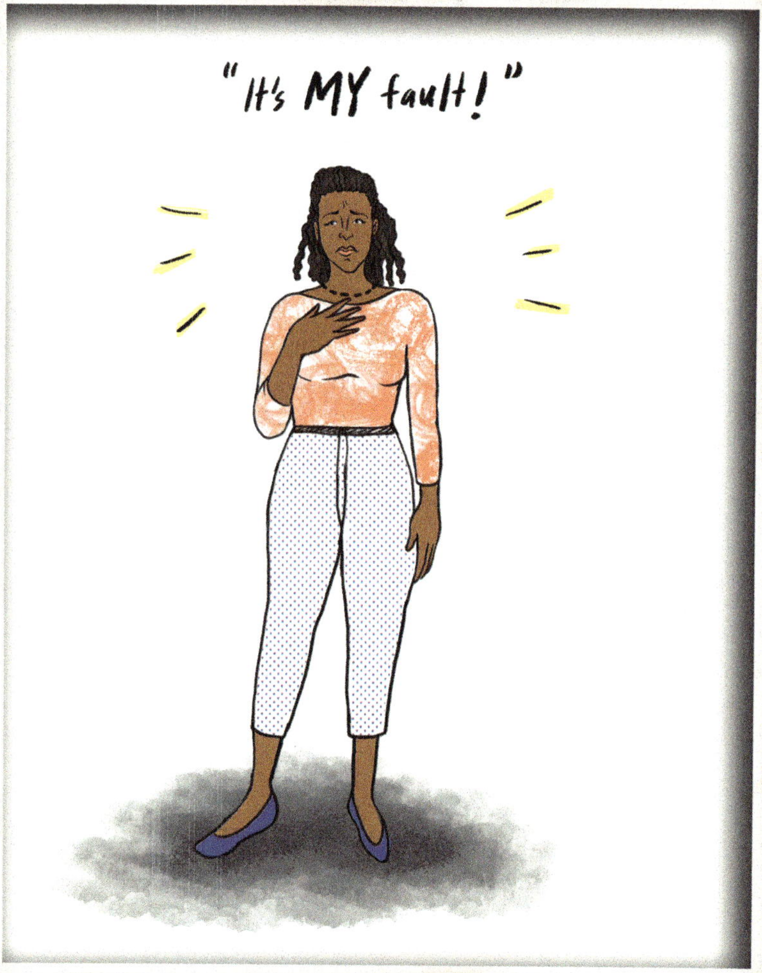
"It's MY fault!"

Chapter XII:
Life with Others

The First Rite

Naming Ceremonies

Rites of Passage are ritualized in all cultures. The naming ritual, for example a christening or a bris, not only identifies the infant with a name but also introduces him into his cultural and extended family. He is given his own unique spot. The extended family and community is solicited for support and solace, both for him and his parents who are all now accepted as part of the collective community. This support and solace can be especially helpful during the fog of the early weeks.

Entering the Spirit World

Giving an infant a name not only identifies him as an individual separate from his parents; but, at the same time, it incorporates him into his community and into the spirit world of that culture: To make this infant part of the supporting community, some Western Christian cultures will commonly name an infant after a saint who lives eternally within the religion. In the Jewish religion, an infant is often named after a relative who has passed away. The relative is thus never forgotten and lives on in this new little person. While the infant becomes an individual, he or she also remains part of the culture, and of the spirit of this flowing humanity.

Emerging into one's culture

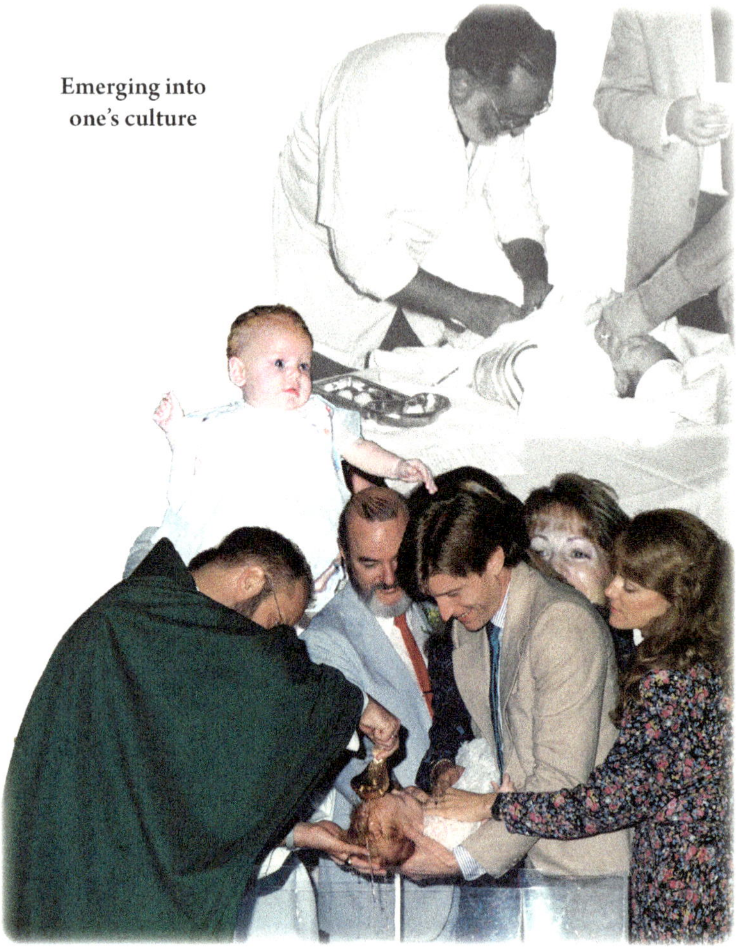

But at the same time, parents often try hard to further individualize the child by giving him a unique nickname, one that, with hope, no other parent has ever used.

The Navajo Laughing Ceremony

Perhaps one of the more interesting naming ceremonies is the Navajo Laughing Ceremony. The Navajo Indians do not give an infant a name until he has his first laugh. This usually occurs around three months of age. The momentous event is celebrated with a big party. But...whoever evoked the first laugh must bring all the food! As one can imagine, this is a great way to keep many visitors away during the early weeks. It is interesting to note that the infant does not receive a name of his own until he has laughed or behaved like a separate, outgoing, social little person.

Conflicting Advice, Revisited

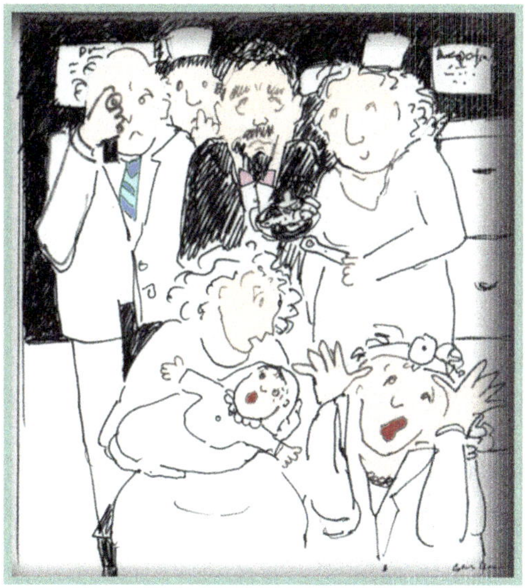

"Isn't there one right way?

Having a growing newborn or infant invites everyone else's so-called expertise. Others are more than willing to offer their advice with pride and confidence. They have survived this rite of passage, know all about it, and now want to give sage advice on how to survive. This phenomenon materializes, I am sure, in all cultures and countries. In the United States, even strangers in a grocery store feel entitled to give advice (see "*Everybody is Entitled to My Opinion*," in Chapter I). In other countries, like Sweden, this public "stranger" advice would hardly be dreamed of. Maternity advice in many other world cultures is more often than not given primarily in the "red tent" part of that culture, not by strangers in the grocery store. But rest assured it takes place somehow and somewhere in all cultures.

Of course, there is rarely one "right way" to raise children. Each parent comes from different backgrounds with different ghosts; each child has a different temperament; different socioeconomic backgrounds exist, and different physical problems come into play. Different answers exist to multiple problems. From the perspective of a chef, there are myriad different recipes for making bread, none of which is right or wrong. So, what are parents to do when they seek advice?

"My advice" (I say this with a smile) is to stick to one advisor, which will help to avoid conflicting advice. One nurse may recommend trying A, B, C. Another may recommend B, A, C. It does not mean that one is right and the other is wrong; it simply means there are different ways to approach the issue, just as there are indeed different ways of making bread. Stick with one trusted source, whether that is your pediatrician, nurse, lactation consultant, or doula; filter all the advice through that person. Sport professionals have their own coaches, not several different coaches for the same thing. So pick one coach, one chef, one expert that you trust. Also rely on your own observations, judgments, and instincts, which will help to enhance your own observational powers and sense of confidence. Then bounce your thoughts off your coach. You will even seek advice throughout the Internet. Now that can be conflicting. So then again, bounce your thoughts off your coach. That's "my advice!"

Guilt, Blame, and Me

Guilty of Guilt

Getting out of the fog of these feelings involved in the early weeks requires dealing with guilt.

Guilt is complex. It's ubiquitous. All normal loving parents are at some point captured by guilt. Constant, obsessive questions insert themselves into the everyday enjoyment of having this infant. *"Am I doing this right?" "Am I dressing him well enough for the weather?" "Am I talking with him enough?" "Am I doing enough for everyone? My mother is coming to visit. My husband is alone. What do I do?"* (See the anecdote *"Trying to Please Everyone, But Not Harry,"* in the Prequel.)

Sometimes guilting yourself is not acceptable; "it" (whatever the issue may be) must become someone else's fault. To a spouse you might say, *"Why don't you help me?"* To a relative, *"Why are you so judgmental?"* These are automatic and magical attempts to relieve your own burden of guilt. It is as if those other people are creating the problem. This projection of your guilt onto others can allow you to feel less apparent stress: *"It's their fault, not mine; I'm not personally responsible for this, they are."* (See "Projection" in the glossary.)

And Then There Is Always an "I"

To get a handle on guilt and guilting, one ***must*** absolutely understand its origin. Nothing else works! Reassurance from others fails. Sympathy and attempts to comfort the guilty party fail. Rationalizing fails. Blaming fails. Guilt will simply reoccur and reoccur. There is just no other way to handle it. You must understand the power in the seed that gives birth to guilt. There is no other way to conquer it.

Ok, so where does it come from?

"Listen to the words!" insisted an elder psychoanalyst to a small group of young doctors feeling constant guilt as they dealt with dying pediatric cancer patients dropping around them in the old days. (His research into guilt was later published in the *New England Journal of Medicine* in the 1970s.) When you listen to expressions of guilt, what do you hear?

Listen.

Wait.

Simply listen.

...Listen to the words.

Listen...

No! Wait! Simply open your mind and quietly and calmly listen ...

> *"It's **my** fault; **I** should not have done that." Or, "**I** should have done that instead." "Am **I** doing this right?" "What else can **I** do to stimulate this baby?" "How can **I** make him happy?" "**I** should not have taken him out in this weather!"*

There is always an "*I*." Perhaps that is why we capitalize the letter; it is all about "***Me***."

*"Did **I** bring him in too late (to the doctor); would it have made a difference?" "What am **I** doing wrong?"* And it goes on and on, and on and on, and on and on! In Ingmar Bergman's famous 1957 classic film *Wild Strawberries,* the professor was told in his dream, ***"You are guilty of guilt!"***

Yes, in fact it is your fault.

Yep! That's right. It is indeed your fault for feeling guilty.

Wait a minute, you're supposed to make me/us feel good in this book!

I'm trying, just listen. Hang on!

Guilt makes us feel good.

What?

Yep. It makes us powerful, really powerful: *"It's my fault. I should have been* (powerful enough) *able to fix it."*

Wow!

It's all about "me." "I" should have been powerful enough to protect, prevent, fix.

Well, are we that powerful, or do we wish we were that powerful?

Can we stop maladies; can we fix all problems; can we make everyone, all our children, our spouse, all our relatives happy all the time? Can we prevent our children from ever stumbling and falling? Can we take every stone off their path? Can we prepare a perfectly smooth journey to their future and guarantee success at every turn? If we can't maybe it is someone else who is failing to help?

Guilt helps us live with our failed wishes for the problems of reality, and yet still feel powerful and in control. It's the *"should have been."* In other words, when something goes awry we *"should have been"* able to prevent it; we *"should have been"* that powerful.

But we weren't! And that's the hook.

We are not above life and reality. We are not God. We are not "all-powerful."

Yet **we live an illusion thinking we are**, or should be, in control all the time when, in fact, we are not. We think we can prevent errors, mistakes, and avoid all problems if we but practice to perfection, do the right thing, read the right books, and avoid the pitfalls.

And who wants to give up that illusion?

In reality, none of us! That's why it is hard to conquer guilt! Why in the world would I want to feel, or recognize, helplessness?

Well, we are not helpless; but we are not all powerful either. We simply do the best we can and that is the best we can do. Maybe we are just not as powerful as we wish we were. Accepting that is not an easy pill to swallow!

Guilt causes pain; preoccupation with it can actually inhibit one from a desired goal. It can be self-defeating. If we are preoccupied with guilt we are thinking that we are above reality; we are not accepting our own human limits. So, it is worth working on; it is worth accepting reality. We are not above reality. We may think/wish things were our fault; then we could have fixed them. But they may not be; and, even when they were, it is a reality that we are not superhuman and capable of a mistake-free existence. Better to take these experiences as opportunities to learn and keep on going. Life is not all about me and what I could have done.

Guilt is all about Ego

You should have been so strong. Or if it is not you and your fault, then it must be someone else's fault. Someone should be responsible, someone must be larger than life.

Alas, perhaps we have to come down to earth. No one is sufficiently powerful to make everything perfect. Thus, we must give up that wish to be all-powerful, that wish that we could have made the difference. Only by understanding and accepting the origins of guilt will you be able to master guilt, feel more comfortable, and actually have a chance to achieve more without guilt's often very heavy burden.

Guilt makes me important! Again, **guilt is all about ego**. *"I'm always worried that I'm not doing enough. Am I hurting Harry by giving into all his needs? Sometimes he gets bored, and I feel I must entertain him."* Guilt makes me the hub of the wheel, the center of attention, the most important. And again, who wants to give that up? It's tough to realize, to face, that life is not all about me.

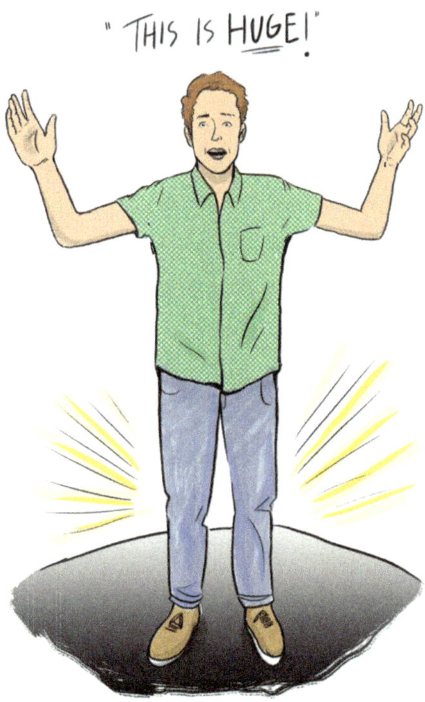

But to feel relief and to be even more efficient and effective, one must actually consciously strive to give up that feeling of being all-important. You are important, you are powerful. You are just not all-powerful and you are not the only important person. *"Already, I'm too tough on myself."* (See the beginning anecdote *"Trying to Please Everyone, but Not Harry."*)

Give yourself a break! Don't be so tough on yourself. You can't do it all; it's simply not possible. So give it up! **Let it go!**

But that is hard, even for the least of us: I once heard someone say, *"I may not be much, but I'm all I think about!"*

You have to share your responsibilities. You have to depend on others. You must at times trust and be forgiving. You just can't do it all by yourself and you can't be perfect. You have to come down to Earth and be with the rest of us. **We all are just not larger than life.**

It's also about the First Law of Thermodynamics:

Energy can neither be created nor destroyed but it changes forms and can flow from one place to another.

So, if you can relinquish that sometimes-enormous energy used on yourself for maintaining guilt, that energy can then be used more efficiently, to not make as many guilt/anxiety-distracted errors, and to move onto putting it into warm, deep, enjoyable feelings with creative love expressions for your new thrilling family!

Now that is HUGE (again)!

Guilt, by the way, is not the same as concern and worry. Also, interestingly, an unbelievable magical part to guilt exists but that is another story, perhaps for Book III. For now, **on to control and magic.**

Fears and Magic

Worry and Love

Is there a new parent who does not have fears? Is there a new—or even experienced—parent who does not worry? **An axiom repeated: Once you love, you worry.** You are doomed to worry. Once you love someone, you worry. We worry about a healthy pregnancy and then a healthy delivery. That is supplanted quickly with worries of adequate growth and feeding. Soon those worries are followed by, "How do I prevent misfortune?" But one must keep some perspective in one's worries.

Discovering ways to avoid danger can alleviate worries. For example, SIDS can be prevented, to a large extent, by having an infant sleep on its back. But try as we may to avoid problems, **we still reach beyond reality and into magic**, into miraculous ways to help us in this fight:

The Evil Eye

Hardly a culture exists that does not have and dread at least some concept of "The Evil Eye" in some form or another. The Evil Eye is particularly prevalent in Mediterranean and Middle Eastern cultures. The omnipresent Evil Eye remains forever vigilant.

If one dares prepare with excitement and joyous anticipation for the coming newborn, the infant may be born with some punishing malady. If, after birth, he is handsome and content, a parent is apprehensive about feeling happiness without fearing that the Evil Eye may punish by inflicting the infant with colicky misery. If one's infant is healthy, there should be no rejoicing, not even momentarily. If there is jubilation, something foreboding may descend upon the infant. Common phrases are *"Don't jinx it," "Don't tempt fate."* The parent or family may be damned with illness or failure, for the Evil Eye is always watching. Thus a parent's young, naive, presumptuous delight, or a proud or boastful expression, may have the power to cause illness. A parent or infant may be punished by the Evil Eye for that disrespectful frivolity.

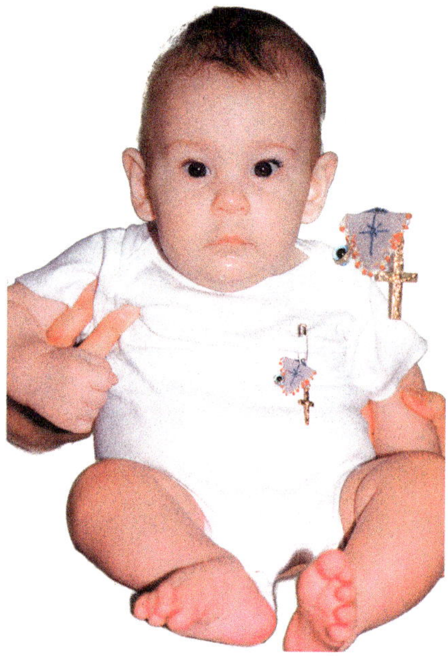

The Cross and the Evil Eye

Amulets

To lovingly protect their/our children, parents embrace magical thoughts and amulets as tangible and concrete representations that empower them to guard their children from evil-eye induced maladies. Magically empowered amulets, medals, or talismans of some sort are worn around the neck to ward off punitive harm from the powerful Evil Eye. East Asians hang jade carvings of Kwan Yin (also Kuan Yin and Guanyin), the "Goddess" of Compassion around the child's neck. Greeks and others from Mediterranean cultures wear jewelry with porcelain Evil Eyes and/or the Greek filigree crosses. Africans have pouches with herbs and remedies to ward off evil. Catholics around the world have "Sacred Heart" badges, scapulars, and Saint Christopher medals. These talismans often arrive as wonderful gifts in silver, gold, and jade from friends and relatives.

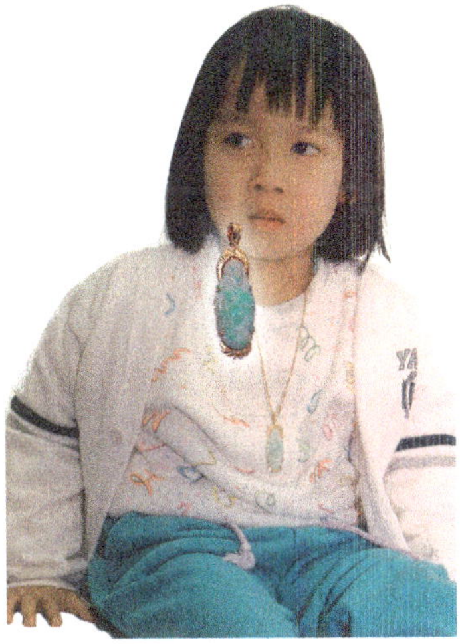

The "Goddess" Kwan Yin

Many cultures also embrace the magically protective concept of "knocking on wood": *"If I do dare express gratefulness for my infant's health, I can protect him from my sin of pride if I but knock on wood immediately after saying it!"* Some people, after expressing some positive feature concerning their child, will exclaim, *"Thank God!"* while simultaneously using the crooked index finger of their right hand to "knock on wood."

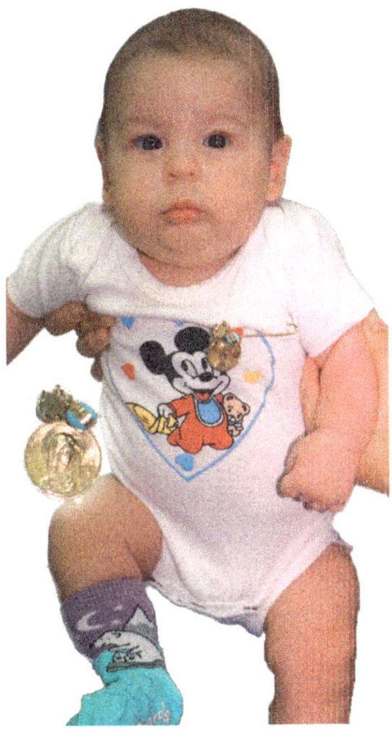

The Virgin Mary & The Evil Eye

Islam not only has the Evil Eye; they also have their own protective incantation: *Insha'Allah. Insha'Allah* or "God willing" is a powerful mantra of protection. A more powerful incantation also exists: *"Masha' Allah."* This incantation magically protects the child from the Evil Eye who will punish the child with illness or malady because of the Evil Eye's justified wrath toward the parents for any glee they might have for their child's health, development, or good looks. Some cultures further protect the delivery of a healthy child by avoiding preparations, even forbidding Western culture baby showers. They don't want to "jinx" it.

Scandinavian cultures have another variation of the Evil Eye concept. In fact, it has been incorporated into everyday behavior. While having few amulets they do have protective jewelry with Christian crosses. But daring to express praise or pride for themselves or their children may condemn them to failure. Indeed, to feign shyness and humility is lauded, perhaps to a fault. A common Swedish expression is, *"One's own praise smells bad."* Swedes are also often seen "knocking on wood."

The Evil Eye guarantees retribution for happy or thankful feelings and engenders guilt in us for even having those feelings. **Thus, amazingly, by believing in the Evil Eye and by feeling guilty about a happy or thankful feeling, we become powerful!**

What!?

Yep, we feel we can ward off the retribution of the Evil Eye if we but punish ourselves ahead of time and feel bad about being thankful that we have a healthy infant: **That way nothing bad will happen.** Thus, **the incantations and amulets bestow us with magical power, a feeling of being in control**. Also, talismans become symbolic, visible ways that empower us to protect our child. While we may not be that powerful, the amulet and/or incantation is. We ourselves thus avoid the guilt that may come our way if something bad were to happen. We did everything we could; we attached the evil eye amulet on the child. And we can tell our forebears. So, should something happen, they cannot blame us. We again did everything we could.

It is very hard to accept that in reality we are simply just not that powerful. While the amulet or incantation fulfills our wish to protect, it does nothing other than to make us feel we have done everything we can. In reality, it cannot ward off maladies and misfortune. We have to do that, to the best of our ability. But then life still throws hard things our way. The problem is that we are not God; we are just not powerful enough to have everything perfect with no problems, no glitches whatsoever. Now who wants to accept that? And so, we may continue to reach beyond reality and into magic to attempt grasping for perfection with unquenched happiness.

The Other Side of Magic, Rites...and Guilt

Amulets and Incantations

All the above being said, many, if not most in the world, obviously feel truly protected and/or empowered by incantations and talismans. That is completely respected. Amulets and incantations may also mean "Best Wishes." They can be friendly, magical gifts from well-wishers. These offerings are part of the culture. What's wrong with that?

Absolutely nothing... in my mind. Perhaps some iconoclasts may put them down. But I personally think talismans, after understanding their traditional meaning, are wonderfully acceptable tangible, culturally derived thoughts for wishing one well, or one's child well. They may also be friends' and relatives' expressions of love with their wishes to join in the protection of this new, vulnerable infant.

When I'm not a fan is if these kinds of gifts are used forebodingly, ominously portending some future misfortune causing dread, if they are not embraced. Parents already have it hard enough, and need not any further unnecessary worries.

Rites of Passage

Now onto more magic, that seen and marveled at in the rituals around Rites of Passage.

Magic and rituals can be fun. We are curious about them and love to watch and/or participate in our own as well as in those of others' cultures. Rites of Passage involve age-old, often centuries-old rituals that help all the different members of a culture or group adjust to the change of the individual(s) as he/she separates from one group to join (or intrude into) another. The ritual validates the change and helps all accept the loss/separation from the first group and intrusion into the new group.

Two examples follow: one from the end of childhood, and one at its beginning.

Graduation from college (or high-school, or any school) is formally and portentously celebrated at college's end. Seriously traditional gowns and caps of old adorn ceremonious parades, along with music. Importuning, advise-giving speeches precede acceptance of certifications.

The ceremony honors the one graduating to impress him (or her) with the realization that he is leaving the ofttimes frivolous student life to purportedly step into the world of grown-ups, and to seek now, on his own, the status either of a self-sufficient job or further specialized adult education.

But the ritualized Rite is not just for the individual. It is also for those he is leaving, helping them to let go and accept him as an adult. And it is for those whom he is joining: He can't just barge (intrude) into that world and declare himself as a well-educated adult. He must be certified to be considered capable of joining their ranks.

In the various "naming" ceremonies (for examples: the bris, baptism, or "laughing" ceremonies), the newborn leaves the world of yearning to be delivered as a reality upon the face of the earth. His presence is commanding and intrudes into the existing relationships of his parents, other siblings if they exist, and his relatives. The parents, friends, and relatives celebrate this arrival, which soothes the intrusion. A name is given so the intrusion arrives as an undeniable person requiring respect and acceptance. He is now here, and must be dignified with deference by all as a reality with a real name. He is now part of the culture. He will be loved (just as you are loved). And so, the naming ceremonies are ritualized, becoming repetitive cultural templates not only to welcome these new ones upon this earth and into their cultures but also to aid those already here in adjusting to that intrusion.

That is the true beauty, the magic, the rich feeling-color, and color we marvel at with awe in the rituals of the Rites of Passage.

Guilt

Now to guilt: Some may say that a person, committing offense, should indeed feel some guilt. If guilt were simply thoughtful worry and concern that led to self-improvement, that would be great. But pure guilt feeling, besides being "all about me," may also be a magical method to actually **avoid the exertion** necessary for thoughtful, beneficial, action-oriented change to rid oneself more permanently of the offending behavior.

What?

Well more on this in another, perhaps the next, book.

He

loves

her !

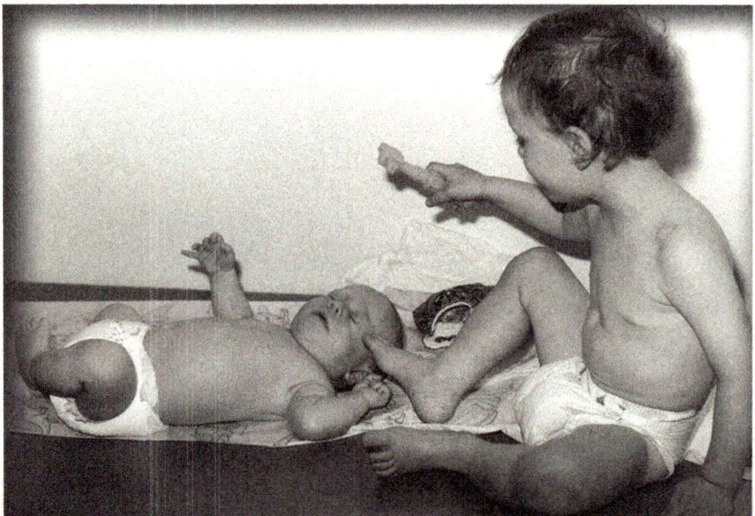

Chapter XIII: Dealing with the Little One

The Older Ones

One mother recounted the following about a three-year-older sister:

"She's great with her [the new arrival].
She loves to read to her.
I just wish she wouldn't sit on her when she does it."

A clever little tip for this is to have a playpen (or a "pack-and-play") in the most common living space, like the kitchen. You can usually obtain one at a really low price at a yard sale, Goodwill, or online. When you are together in the common space but preoccupied with a chore like cooking, you can put the new baby in the pack-and-play. It is like having a little safety fence around the baby for protection. It's great to maintain separation between a newborn and older siblings and pet dogs. And you don't have to be vigilant for absolutely every second. Moreover, the fence being in place means you are not the one who must push the sibling, or the pet, away thus causing them to have hurt feelings of exclusion.

It's a great idea to prepare older siblings as is described in Book I. But no matter how much you prepare them for a new arrival you are, with all the new preoccupations and work, just simply not going to be as available as you were before. You won't be able to dote on your older one as much as before. There is just not that much time in the day. So, they will feel that! Initially, it is not so much sibling rivalry that is felt; it is just simply missing you.

You anticipate that and thoughtfully deal with it with **empathy**. Try to keep some scheduled time alone together, even if it is but fifteen minutes. Set a timer or draw a picture of a timer that can represent the time you will get together. Let them know that you feel the same way. When you are engrossed in small infant care, tell them to hang in there; soon you will have that special time together. Meanwhile, let them watch a video of yourselves together that you created during pregnancy (see Book I).

Infant Clues and Parent Detectives

Is It Physical, or Is It Temperament?

Understandably, given obvious inexperience, neophyte parents are often clueless. To cope in navigating through the initial fog, parents are forced into becoming detectives.

Think about what it must be like to be an infant: You can't scratch that itch. You are stuck in a baby body that can't do what you want it to do. It's hard work to do anything. Your brain is always working faster than your body. You complain with frustration and your startle reflex jerks you out of control, which is hugely frustrating especially if you have a high-strung, easily irritated temperament. Not to mention the fact that you can't communicate your specific needs and discomforts other than through ambiguous crying.

Parents, as a result, must figure out what your current grievance is all about—a real challenge for novice parents intent upon making you happy and calm. So they change your wet diaper, feed you, hold you, and rock you until they find something that works.

For novice parents a very large challenge is sorting out whether the baby's complaints are physical in nature or just a minor irritation or frustration being expressed by an intense temperament. Determining your newborn's temperament can be very reassuring in moments of anxiety when such complaints arise. For help in determining your infant's temperament, see Book I for the TENP scale.

It is not easy for novice parents to discern the different infant cries: Is it a slight irritation? Is it hunger? Is it anger? Is it frustration? Is it pain? It takes time for parents; but eventually they learn the meaning behind the different cries. And they can rely on others who are more experienced to help them sort out the different cries ... sometimes. This usually takes about three months with the first born.

Soothing

Book I has descriptions and photos of several very effective soothing techniques for the newborn. Parents can also discover additional soothing skills specific to their newborn.

The Plug

"What do you think of pacifiers?" parents ask.

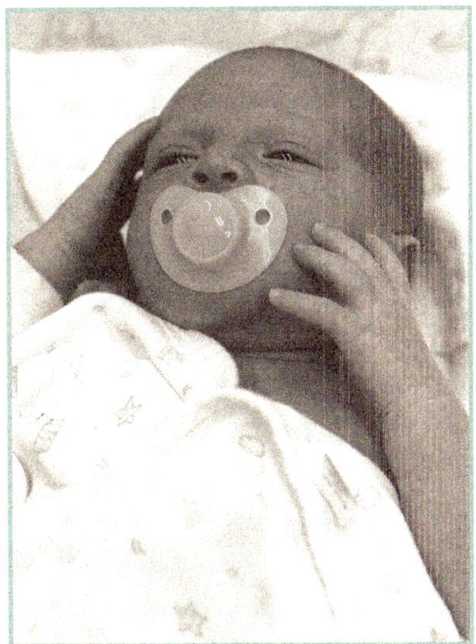

The Plug

Most soon-to-be-new parents do not like the idea of pacifiers because they recall seeing a five-year-old with the pacifier hung on a string around his neck in the grocery store. It's important to remember that most newborns have a strong need to suck. Thus, using a pacifier during this period may be necessary to calm the child. It is also fine to use your little finger (upside down in the roof of his mouth) as a pacifier.

When it comes to pacifiers, some have concerns regarding "nipple confusion."

If your child is mellow he will likely accept anything without complaint.

If your infant is or tends toward high-strung, he may quickly and easily go for the nipple of the bottle, and refuse the breast. The high-strung newborn sees this as a quick fix, an easy resolution of his intolerance of frustration.

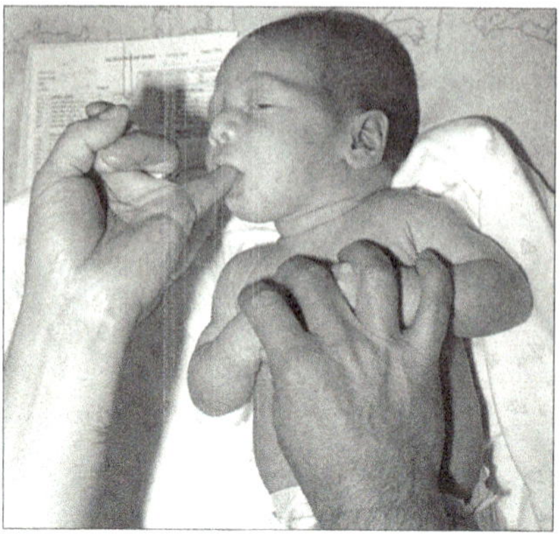

Notice the vigorous sucking

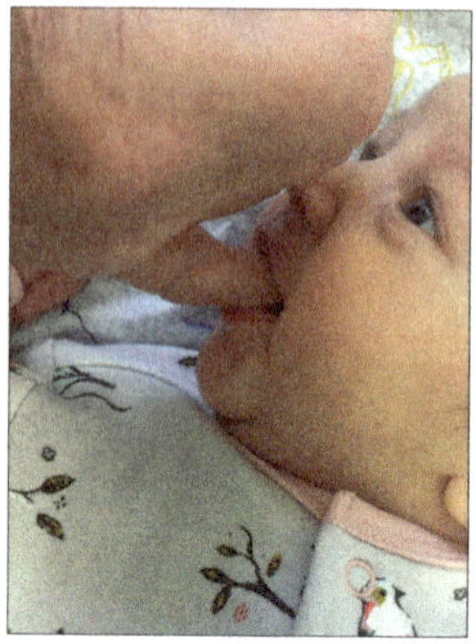

A dysfunctional suck. Notice the open mouth with little sucking due to confusion.

It is also easier for us to push a bottle nipple through the sometimes strongly clinched jaw of this high-strung newborn. However then, this type of infant does not learn the required task of initially relaxing his jaw before latching on to the breast. Breast-feeding may thus quickly become much more difficult for these infants to master. So, if one wants to successfully breast-feed, it's best during the initial weeks to not expose these infants to a pacifier, the nipple of a bottle, or even your upside-down little finger. Thus, with avoiding "nipple confusion," they learn to latch onto the breast.

If these high-strung infants need supplements with formula for excess weight loss, failure to grow, jaundice, or low blood sugar, they may be "cup fed" using little flexible medicine cups to avoid their sucking on the nipples of bottles (See a picture of these cups on page 165 in Chapter XI). Lactation consultants can be very helpful in offering techniques and support. Thus, the infant can learn to eventually relax his jaw to continue breast-feeding without becoming confused by the nipple of the bottle.

So instead of a pacifier, you can offer them the crooked knuckle of your little finger to suck on as a pacifier. This crooked knuckle, unlike the tip of your finger, requires the same suck as the suck needed for the nipple/areola of a breast. This crooked knuckle pacifier also helps the high-strung infant learn how to relax his jaw before he starts to suck on the knuckle. This is the same task he must learn for the breast. So, he can practice and complain while doing so on your crooked knuckle without developing "nipple confusion." Consider this as "Occupational Therapy" for this type of newborn.

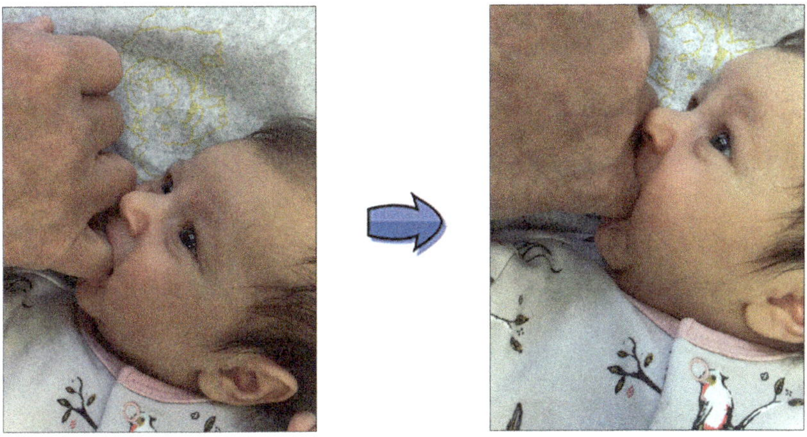

"Occupational Therapy" To Avoid "Nipple Confusion"
Sometimes you must push the jaw down to push the crooked 5th finger knuckle past the clinched jaw. Notice he has a firmer suck (See image on right as compared to the sucking seen in the image on the left) when the crooked finger is past the dysfunctionally clinched jaw. If you use the nipple of a bottle, an upside-down finger, or a pacifier, he will have a difficult time learning to latch onto the breast. But sucking on the crooked knuckle requires the same sort of suck as on the nipple/areola of the breast and helps him to learn how to relax his jaw clinching reflex.

Empathically Talking to Him

As strange as this sounds, you can actually talk quietly, softly, and empathetically to your complaining newborn; and he will respond by calming down.

Try this: Put him in a sitting position on any table propped up with your hands like crutches in his armpits. Have your head lower than his and respond with a very soft, low voice and with emotionally empathic facial expressions, showing him you identify with his concerns. He will actually cooingly talk (or softly cry/complain) back to you as you gently and empathically talk him down from his concerns. You can share his feelings by saying, *"I know, I know. It's tough being a little kid. You can't scratch your itches; you can't even tell me where they are. I know, I know. It's tough."*

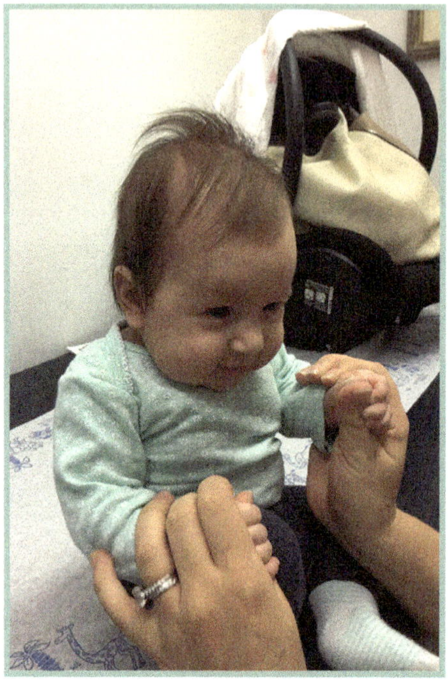

"Hi big guy!
How're you doing?"

The Smoothie

One grandmother to me stated the obvious: Touch is soothing. She called the following technique a "smoothie": This is essentially a soft, feather-touching massage of the infant's whole body and face and cheeks. This was especially effective when the infant was in her arms in the "Airplane" position, the most soothing position for any infant.

Other Calming Techniques

An infant needs support to handle frustration. See Book I for many more details on newborn temperament and specific calming techniques.

Can You Spoil a Baby?

"I have heard you can't spoil a baby."

"Is it true you should never let a baby cry?"

"My husband says, 'Let him cry a little.' But I just can't do that. My own mother says you can't let a baby cry."

"Dr. Sears and his wife say you should never let a baby cry."

What Does "Spoil" Mean?

This, perhaps the most common first conflict between parents, is one of the nicest and one of the most loving because both parents want their baby happy; they just differ in the approach. So, let's look at it.

What does "spoiling" mean, and does age matter?

In my mind "spoiling a child" means that the infant or child would have been indulged with excessive kindness or pampering to the extent that he is unhappy living with the frustrations of life because he has to wait to see if someone else will solve them for him. It's a matter of time and petulance. It is sort of simple, I think: If the child learns to handle his own frustrations, he does not have to wait around petulantly for someone else to do it for him. He can do it himself, and do it when he wants it done. He makes himself happy; and he learns self-mastery and that he need not remain dependent upon someone else to do something/whatever for him to make him happy. He does not have to wait for the solution; he solves it himself. But a baby? Can we expect that of a baby?

What's the Goal?

Answer: Clearly, happiness and contentment.

But the problem is that they have just jumped out of the snuggly womb and literally landed on the planet. They breathe the air, **so now they can cry**. They are no longer swaddled in the womb. On our planet, their arms fling out in the startle reflex, which drives them crazy since they are in no control of that reflex. We can take over and swaddle them and perform all the other calming techniques described in Book I. But they must learn themselves; they have to push themselves to master those reflexes and the planet's gravity to progress to intentionally reaching out and touching you, to concentrate on smiling at you, to coo and talk with you. You can't just smile for them; it doesn't work that way. **They are the ones who must learn those things**. They must do it themselves and it begins when confronted with the gravity of the planet upon exiting the womb. But we can help them. And there is the conflict: how and how much, and when?

Learning starts after birth. **Imitation** is one way to learn. As an example, if a parent repeatedly sticks out his or her tongue, the newborn will quickly learn to imitate that motion in response to the parent's encouragement. A newborn also learns from **causality**: If I am hungry and cry, they will pick me up and feed me, or figure out what is irritating me. The third and very important way of learning is through **frustration-resolution**. A newborn or small infant may have the desire, for example, to simply lift his head up while lying on his stomach. The time between the wish to do this and the accomplishment of the feat is filled with frustrating attempts and complaints. However, when this simple task is accomplished, he feels excitement, a thrill! That excitement, that thrill from the accomplishment is part of a feedback loop. Seeking that thrill, anticipating that reward draws the child into more easily taking on the next frustrating task. Learning to master this method of learning is very important later for evolving toward self-initiated learning (as opposed to "spoon-fed" learning).

Another point here is that your newborn's genetic temperament plays a major role in "frustration tolerance." The mellow newborn hardly complains with these efforts while the high-strung infant can appear furious. The frustration fury of the intense child's temperament may be misread, even intimidating. Their furious frustration can be seen as pain. Or we can become furious with them when they are trying to learn how to breast-feed and their infant reflexes dominate and infuriatingly confound this learning process. We try to rescue and rescue; and it is still difficult. Book I has helpful hints in guiding the high-strung newborn to learn breast-feeding.

Rescue versus Empathy

Let's back up.

For the newborn and infant in the early months, initiating the process of learning is first the desire to do something, for example challenging gravity by just lifting his own head off the mattress. Then with practice, work, and time he gets there. And then the thrill. The actual time interval between the wish and the accomplishment is filled with frustration. So he complains. He cries with frustration, or screams if he is high-strung.

Then the dilemma: Do we just pick him up every time he cries?

If we were to really pick him up with every cry, he may never reach the thrill of accomplishment. He may become dependent on your "rescue" from his frustration before he reaches the thrill. He then learns he has to wait for you to resolve his frustration. You wish him happiness and therefore rescue. But, in fact, the result of your rescue is that he has to wait for you to actually rescue. He has to (learns to) wait for you and seldom realizes that a thrill of accomplishment may be in his future.

So, do we never rescue? You might think, *"If I don't rescue him, he'll feel abandoned."* But there is another approach rather than just total rescue: That is empathy...empathy together with what I call **"a reluctant rescue!"**

Newborns and infants are, for the most part, completely dependent on others to meet their needs. They must be nurtured and they **must** be "rescued." Some parents want to mainly rescue, and to rescue immediately. A spouse may then tend to balance that with an alternate overreaction saying, *"Let him handle it."* But a compromise may be possible, a wise mixture of both: What you can do is to lean over and **empathize**, saying to your infant, *"Come on, you're doing great, you're gonna get there."* But then if it is too hard, you rescue him by picking him up for soothing. You eventually put him back down and say, ***"Go for it."*** But each time you repeat this effort, take just a few seconds longer than the previous time before you rescue him again.

So, to repeat a description of this approach: If the newborn infant is simply fussing as he tries to lift his head, initially empathize with him but rescue him if he finds it impossible. With each following effort, just take one to two seconds longer before you rescue. In other words, you lovingly "**reluctantly rescue.**" Remember, you are not asking him to suddenly go off to college or get a job; you are simply helping him to master the little task of lifting his head off the mattress! It is analogous to learning how to ride a bike later in childhood. Only the child can ride the bike, so you help him and empathize with him as he achieves and feels the thrill of the accomplishment. With the newborn/early infant it is the same for just lifting his head. Only he can lift his head from the mattress; you can't do it for him. Help him toward that simple mastery. Empathizing, soothing, and helping the infant toward self-mastery are far from abandonment. You are not abandoning him; in fact, it is the opposite; you are joining him and forming a team. It's like "spotting" in gymnastics; you safely help them but less and less until they have accomplished it completely themselves. It is then their accomplishment, their thrill!

To do this infant "spotting," parents must ask themselves what is reasonable to expect and then gently help the infant toward that goal despite the infant's understandable frustration. For example, it is quite logical to expect a small infant to be on his tummy for a bit of time while he is awake. This "tummy time" is the position from which lifting his head, rolling over, and crawling are accomplished. So, each time a parent puts the infant down, he can be placed on his stomach, if awake. He may start to fuss, cry, and even become hysterical if high-strung, as he tries to simply lift his head. That is when you empathize, be close, and say soft, encouraging things.

Somewhere between fussing-a-little-bit and crying, but before he becomes hysterical, a parent can calm him down and even help him onto his back or pick him up for a soothing hug. Regardless of the reaction, a parent should still initially put the infant on his stomach at times. Slowly, the infant will fuss less and eventually accept and master this position. In this situation, the fathering "role" is crucial in helping the mother (who has symbiotic feelings) survive their infant's apparent unhappiness. It is worth noting that the different parenting roles, while gender-related, are not gender-specific. In other words, some fathers can have symbiosis and take on the mothering role, and some mothers can take on the fathering role. This also applies to m/m and f/f parents. This is a parenting partnership. More on this will be discussed in Book III.

Over the course of twenty to thirty years of growing up, the pendulum for parents should then swing from total rescue for a newborn to empathy with far, far less rescue for grownup children. Parents want their children to be happy. But if they continue to rescue their children from all sources of frustration, the children will expect to be rescued; they will be "spoiled," expecting or demanding everyone else to do this or that to make them happy. If children eventually learn to master their own frustrations, their problems will often be solved faster and they will be much happier over time.

So, when that infant matures into young adulthood, parents juggle whether to rescue their now adult child from problematic situations (such as paying off credit card debt for a twenty-six-year old son or daughter), or empathize with their adult offspring's challenge (asking what plans might he have for a solution to the debt). In empathizing with their grown-up children, parents aren't abandoning them; rather, they are encouraging them toward self-mastery.

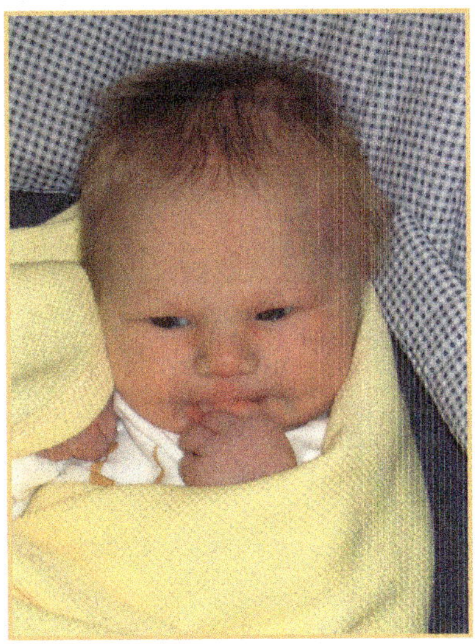

"Go for it! You're doing great!"

Thus, my answer to the question we pediatricians frequently receive about spoiling a baby versus letting him "cry it out" is as follows: As parents, you undoubtedly agree that you want your infant to be happy. Initially, this means totally rescuing him but also empathizing with some of his frustrations (for example, lifting his head or briefly tolerating the irritation of a messy diaper that you are frantically trying to change). Along the way, you help him adapt to life on this planet. You empathize with him as he learns to master life's complexities. You empathetically and softly **"reluctantly rescue."** You expect him to handle a task, such as "tummy time." But before rescuing him, each time you empathize and take just a few seconds longer before you rescue. In this way, you help him as you let him feel the thrill of his own "frustration-resolution," so that he can be happier and more secure in the long run during his journey.

This results, with time, in developing the confidence and security necessary for self-initiated learning. With mastery comes the thrill, which then helps the infant and child feel confident as he seeks the thrill in mastering the next frustration. He also learns that he has not been abandoned in this process; he learns his parent is always there, lovingly empathizing while not necessarily performing an immediate rescue. And he also learns that his parent is there should a caring, albeit slightly reluctant, rescue be necessary. He learns self-confidence. Now, admittedly, this is a two-to-three-decade process. And you are just at the beginning. But it is worth mapping out so you see the future.

What Inhibits Us from Empathy?

You may never, or hardly ever, have experienced it! You yourself may have grown up always rescued; or alternatively you may have grown up feeling abandoned by parents who were actually not there or who were (or were perceived as) emotionally unavailable for whatever reason!

Some parents will still continue to say, *"I'll try but I don't think it will work"* or *"So, you're saying I should just let him cry it out!"* When one hears that question it definitely sounds like there are only two stark choices: "rescue" the infant, or "abandon" the infant to "cry it out." No, there is another way, another repertoire, and that is empathy not abandonment. You join your infant's team; that is not abandonment.

In my experience, this feeling (and this will be discussed in detail in later books) that *"if I don't rescue then I am abandoning my infant/child and I can't do that"* comes from one of two sources: (1) Either the parent has been raised in a total rescue mode by his or her parents, who themselves got into that mode because of a "ghost" in their own parents' nursery. This new parent has thus never experienced the alternative mode of "rescue and empathy," their only repertoire being that of "rescue or abandonment." They have never experienced the loving "empathy" mode. And thus, the rescue-versus-abandonment repertoire is passed on from one generation to the next. Alternatively, (2) this parent has had a loss or an emotionally unavailable parent of her/his own. They are then left with the feeling that *"I don't want you (the infant or child) to ever feel like I felt."* They overcompensate and perpetually rescue. Again, to not rescue feels like abandonment. For them, they are reliving a visceral PTSD. The parents in this situation are actually treating themselves; they are soothing themselves, as they imagine their infant feeling like they felt, for the lost aspects of their own childhood. **Rescue versus Abandonment is a very different repertoire from Rescue versus Empathy.** (More on this will come throughout this book series.)

Parents often comment, *"But it's not good for him to cry and be unhappy and frustrated."* **But frustration is not unhappiness**; it's just frustration. And a little frustration is a necessary part of learning. All parents would agree: we want our infant to be happy, pure and simple. Consider this: If the infant or child or young adult must wait for someone to rescue him from each and every frustration, he must wait longer than if he learns, over time, to solve his own frustrations more quickly when he wishes them to be solved. He can then make himself happier more quickly, and with a sense of security and the thrill of accomplishment. He can actually learn faster if he goes for it himself with that thrill that comes with self-initiated learning. He does not have to wait for someone to teach him everything. And with empathy, support, and encouragement from parents, the infant landing on the planet and now progressing on the path of growing up will never feel a sense of abandonment. **You will always be there when he really needs you! You are now a team!**

Empathy is not sympathy. With sympathy, one simply feels pity or compassion for the other's hardships. But with empathy, one vicariously experiences the emotions and thoughts of someone else. Further, with empathy one feels not only the feelings but passes on, engenders, or encourages a sense of mastery: *"Come on, you're doing great. I know, I know, but you can do it, don't worry. I'm here."* So empathy is more like sympathy but with an empowerment.

It's Still Not Easy

Even if while growing up you have indeed experienced the "empathy" mode it is still difficult to not feel the urge to "rescue" someone you love, especially in the beginning.

Perhaps it is "symbiosis?" Symbiosis is the warm and wonderful merging of feelings between mother and infant whereby the mother feels the infant's feelings as if they were her own. If the newborn has a blood test in the hospital and the mother is present, it is as if she, the mother, is also getting poked with the needle. It is an unstoppable, instinctive, basic gut feeling. So, when an infant is crying, the mother is feeling it herself as if it were her own feeling of pain, frustration, hunger, or whatever source of the crying. The mother's face will often have the identical face of the unhappy newborn or infant.

It does not take a lot of time for the infant to also symbiotically feel the mother's feelings. Most (not all, but most) mothers experience this symbiotic attachment with their newborn and later infant. Some fathers/partners will as well but it is usually part of the maternal "role" during attachment, perhaps evoked from the power of the Biochemistry of Love discussed above. The father's attachment role and the mother's attachment role and their differences are discussed in detail in Book III.

Symbiosis enhances the empathy in the "rescue versus empathy" mode. Symbiosis does not automatically conjure up abandonment feelings. Abandonment feelings come from an instinctive PTSD, from perceived feelings you yourself grew up under. Now this needs pondering if you find yourself in a constant and persistent rescue mode.

Still it is not easy to decide when to empathize and when to rescue. That is a never-ending balancing act. So to decide when to rescue and when to empathize it is helpful to (1) understand the nature of the infant's temperament; (2) realize the difficulty a parent has in helping the infant overcome frustration when the parent is warmly and closely "perceiving" the infant's frustration as unhappiness and as if that unhappiness were the parent's own unhappiness (symbiosis); (3) comprehend the difference between "rescue," "empathy," and "abandonment"; (4) help the infant to adapt to his environment; and finally (5) spook the "ghosts" out of the "nursery." (See "Ghosts in The Nursery" in Chapter III.) In this process, parents should see themselves not only as nurturers but also as **teachers**, helping the infant adapt to his environment, his new world.

That learning process can bring thrill after thrill for you in your own learning process of parenting.

Wish versus Reality...Again

> ***"Reality is a major source of stress...for those who are in touch with it."***
>
> —Lilly Tomlin

"I expected serenity and instead received colic!" lamented one mother. Another mother, who had a high-strung newborn, understatedly uttered, *"Well, I got a little bit more than I had bargained for."*

What I have come to call "Wish versus Reality" involves a concept of conflict, a conflict that inevitably arises between what we really wish to happen versus what actually transpires. Understanding this conflict and its resolution serves us well in coping when reality confronts our everyday wishes for our children.

One of the earliest conflicts involving Wish versus Reality can arrive with delivery. Sometimes the infant's temperament is different from what the parents were expecting. This, the most common expectation, can lead to a thwarted wish with the parent, anticipating a quiet, sweet cuddly baby, instead receiving a high-strung frustration-intolerant newborn. If any drastic difference occurs from what parents' expectations are, an adjustment must be made. During this time an actual mourning process may occur.

Other Wish-Versus-Reality conflicts result if complications occur with the pregnancy or delivery, even if it is a simple variation from normal. Many mothers have the wish and are longing to go home with their baby on the third hospital day. If the reality of breast-milk jaundice intrudes, requiring additional hospitalization, it can be truly saddening for the mother who was expecting to go home. An unanticipated emergency C-section can jolt parents out of their wishes for successful natural childbirth and thrust them into grieving mode. (See "*The Emergency C-section*" and "*A Lower Grade*" in Book I.) Another example is the unanticipated birth of a premature infant (or multiple premature infants). A twin birth is a challenge: A mother may be yearning to bond closely to a single child and, when told she will have twins, wonders how can she love (or manage!) two infants and do as well.

Parents who have been fortunate enough to have most of their wishes fulfilled throughout their lives are going to be the most vulnerable to the disappointments of reality. They may have been brought up protectively, or constantly "rescued" from needing to solve their own disappointments and frustrations by their own overly solicitous parents (See "*The Carefree Socialite*" in Chapter IX.). Others may not have learned, as they themselves grew up, to adapt to their own genetically endowed temperament that inherently compromises their tolerance for frustration. Additionally, some parents may be in positions or professions where they are used to controlling situations and being paid for getting their way.

The Wish versus Reality conflict for parents recurs repeatedly throughout the child's development. Worries arise about their school and social performances, especially when parents' hopes for them are greater than the reality in which the child is growing up. A natural, almost instinctual, compelling feeling exists whereby parents hunger for their children to do well, to have it better, and to do better. Their very understandable investment in their children enhances these parents' own self-worth. Parents yearn for their children to fulfill their own unfulfilled desires. If the child fails to provide a good reflection, parents may then feel disappointment or even anger.

These Wish versus Reality conflicts can be disheartening at best and immobilizing and depressing at worst. When confronted with a Wish versus Reality conflict, acquiescing to reality can be difficult, especially if one wants to effect a change that complies with one's longed-for outcome for the situation. While not easy, one's ability to eventually adapt to reality and give up the wish is determined foremost by one's own temperament and then, subsequently, how that temperament has been nurtured while growing up.

But should a parent complacently accept everything that reality dumps on him or her, or their child? Or should that parent fight to change all that is dumped on him or her? One's first response could be in the form of the common quote: *"It is what it is."*

But perhaps the best answer comes from the now famous Serenity Prayer, its origin actually dating far back and from the Stoic philosopher Epictetus (c. 55–c.135 AD).

The Serenity Prayer

"May I have the serenity to accept the things I cannot change, the courage to change the things I can, and the wisdom to know the difference."

A more light-hearted version for parents comes from the philosopher W. W. Bartley, who in 1961 put the thought together with a Mother Goose rhyme *("For Every Evil...")* from 1695:

"For every ailment under the sun
There is a remedy, or there is none;
If there be one, try to find it;
If there be none, never mind it."

Postface

Research

Western culture's modern family is most often a triad of mother, father, and child, and now partners and child. Some families also exist with a dyad of single parent and child.

When one looks at the amount of research on the usual triad, the majority has been on the mother-child relationship or on just the child or on just the mother; in other words, the research has looked at one side of the triangle. In looking for research on the relationship between father and child and studies on fathers, one observes that the research came later, after a gap was noticed in comparison to studies done on mother and infant. One also observes that the actual quantity of the research on the father-child side of the triangle appears to be less.

Some research exists regarding parenting "roles." Also, anecdotal clinical experience is that most m/m and f/f parents are much like m/f parents in that one usually takes on the "mothering" role with its feelings and the other the "fathering" role and its feelings. Single parents take on both roles and must master the feelings and tasks of both roles. But these "roles" still deal with the mother-child and father-child relationships, again only two sides of the triangle. (More on individual parenting roles will appear in Book III of this series.)

Some research exists regarding the actual psychological development and relationships between the parents, the less obvious third side of the triangle in this parent-child triad. This book, and the series as a whole, further explores that gap in our knowledge of what really happens emotionally and developmentally to husband and wife, partners, as they emerge as a duo after the delivery. To be sure, now they metamorphose and emerge as *father* and *mother*, with new roles and new relationships.

A Truly Important Point

While single parents do not have to deal with The Intruder Complex and f/f parents obviously do not have to deal with "breast feelings" issues, all parents experience love and worry, guilt and guilting, "Wish versus Reality," "Rescue versus Empathy," and other in-common concerns. In other words and simply put, whether we are single, m/f, m/m, or f/f parents, what we all have in common is our children.

And our children change our lives.

The Organization of This Book

To study the relationship between mother and father, the third side of the triangle, one has to look at the whole family and the other points and sides of the triangle and their impact or intrusion, if you will, into that relationship. The child is the third point on the triangle but others from outside the triangle can impact particularly the parent-parent relationship. Like Book I in the series, this book has four sections: The first deals with parents, the second deals with the child, followed by reactions of others, and finally coping concepts.

But that four-section framework may initially seem irritating. For example, in the first section on parents there can be breast-feeding issues and feelings, then in the next section the infant's temperament may impact the breast-feeding, in the third portion others can react to the breast-feeding, and finally in the fourth section coping concepts are offered. One could perhaps put all those together in one topic: breast-feeding from start to finish. But then temperament can impact other areas and not just breast-feeding, and the concepts for coping can be used for other issues, and the reactions of others may not be simply about breast-feeding. If the author went from one topic to the next, we might find coping concepts repeated for each problem. That approach could then be far more nettlesome.

Thus, the above-described format used in this book series means that some repetition of issues will happen, but from different perspectives. The reader might have to be patient when a problem is presented: the answer may appear much later, in the coping concepts part of the book. By putting the coping concepts all together in the final part of the book, parents can perhaps use them for answers to novel problems of their own and on their own.

Attachment Parenting

"Attachment Parenting," espoused in some of the popular baby-book literature lovingly recommends organizing a complementary existence of extended breast-feeding, co-sleeping, "baby wearing," and rescuing. "Rescuing" would be my word for the idea "*that every baby's whimper is a plea for help and that no infant should ever be left to cry*" (*Time Magazine*, May 21, 2012).

I would agree with the initial three recommendations as long as breast-feeding is possible, nourishing, wanted, and enhances bonding and attachment, and if co-sleeping means having the newborn sleep in a bassinet adjacent to the parents' bed and not in the bed with the parents (the latter can be dangerous and is not approved by the American Academy of Pediatrics). However, that fourth approach, I would propose, might veer away from supportive, comfortable attachment into an unhelpful area with unintended and unattuned "rescuing," thus resulting in attachment but possibly a far more worried and less secure attachment.

Every whimper may not be a "plea for help." Some may simply be wonderfully cognitive expressions of frustration, such as when the newborn infant tries to lift his head off the mattress. To say that **every** whimper is a "plea for help" may, in fact, be an imagined projection onto the baby of the parents' experienced feelings from their own childhood, a visceral PTSD if you may. In other words, a parent may have suffered emotional deprivation in his or her own childhood and feel, *"I don't want you to ever feel like I felt."* The parent then imagines, and mistakes, some whimpers of frustration to be instead "pleas for [actual] help."

To let an infant even whimper in frustration might then feel to that parent, actually viscerally, like **abandonment (a PTSD)**. Under these circumstances those new parents appear, in fact, to be reliving their own abandonment from their own childhood. And when that happens, the parent "rescues," even for every whimper. The parents are, in fact, soothing themselves; they are rescuing themselves from their gut memory of their own childhood experience(s).

But there is another mode that I believe is more effective and just as loving, if not more so in a way; one that is far from abandonment; and that is *empathy*. Parents, who have survived an adverse childhood experience(s), or who grew up with parents who rescued constantly because of a "ghost(s) in the nursery," usually and unfortunately have no experience, no repertoire with the mode of empathy unless it is experienced from a relative or later mentor. To give empathy requires, at least, that emotionally available parents or mentors were there for these parents.

This "Rescue vs. Empathy" and other concepts, such as "Wish vs. Reality" and "The Intruder Complex" are detailed in this book (the second in the series). They are, in fact, themes that weave throughout all the books in this series, themes that exist in all of us as parents, perhaps themes that remain immortal.

The Intruder Complex and Growing with Your Child

The divorce rate varies in different cultures. Some countries keep statistics on divorce rates but correct statistics are extraordinarily difficult to obtain. The United States reports a ~50 percent divorce rate. It is said that 10 percent of those marriages ending in divorce are second- and third-time divorces while the remaining 40 percent of the marriages that end in divorce are first-time divorces. Of those first-time divorces in the United States, some have reported that two-thirds occur within six years of the birth of the first child. In Sweden, a while ago, I read a newspaper article that proclaimed a 50 percent divorce rate in that country within the first year of the first child. **Parents, whether divorced or not, remain as parents to their children; there is no escaping that.**

So, it is this author's hope that the dissection of parental feelings will help parents grow with their children. Whether they are married or divorced, they are still parents. For example, it is this author's belief from decades of experience with patients/parents that the Intruder Complex is monumental, nearly universally present, and more often than not unconscious. And, if not dealt with, it can help in or initiate the dissolution of an intact family. That is not to say it is the cause of divorce or uncoupling. If one is looking for the causes for divorce, one must look at the reasons people marry. That is another discussion. However, if the Intruder Complex is recognized and managed, that may help parents to grow along with their children. And would that not be the better for all? Hopefully, its understanding and management will make for happier relationships all around, whether coupled or uncoupled.

How Do We Enjoy All of This?

By understanding what is going on in your relationships, you will be in more control and have more enjoyment of this, the slow rite of passage of parenting.

Relationship problems are ranked as the #1 cause of stress. Thus, Preventive Psychology is what this book series is about. **Yes, it's all about these relationships**: The relationship with yourself and the change in your sense of self, with your partner in this endeavor, the two of you with your child, and then your relationships with others near and around you and your new family.

After any relationship is developed, it settles into a sense of comfort along with some tolerable discomfort. Then another influence, a new presence (for example a child), intrudes from the outside into that or any relationship. A "disturbance" happens and a ripple effect is felt as the intrusion into the relationship creates new changes, changes that force all to adapt in one way or another. There is no avoiding it.

In addition, you enter (or intrude via ritualized templates), mature, and adjust into your family, society, and culture through "Rites of Passage." Your family and society awakens to you: others notice and react. Your own parents are there. Some others help you and celebrate with you, some mentor you, but some compete with you and are less than welcoming.

Thus, the two overarching premises in this book series are that (1) it's all about **relationships and their formation**, and (2) this process of giving birth with its associated parenting also involves **intrusions** into established relationships. Thus, looking at parents through the **prisms** of these two themes, relationships and intrusions, helps explain a lot of the psychological development of parents...and families. And if we can appreciate this development, perhaps we can be more creative teachers of our children. Perhaps we can enjoy it more ourselves and, in the process, help our children feel more security and enjoyment in their lives, and then their children's lives... since now the Ghosts have hopefully been spooked out.

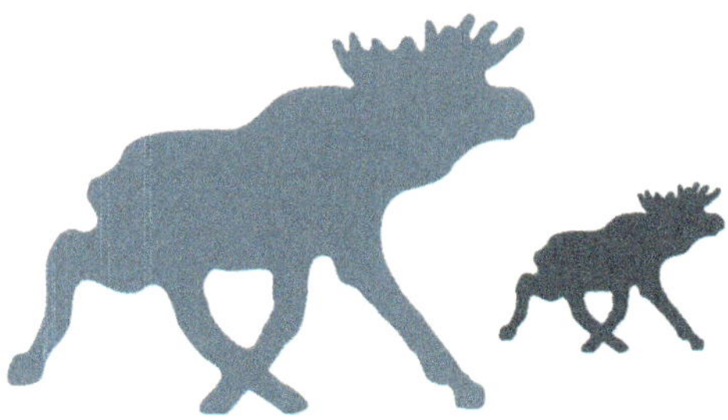

Glossary

Any specialized field, including medicine, often remains esoteric for outsiders because of jargon, argot, abbreviations, and acronyms. When that vocabulary is mastered and understood, the field of interest—in this case pediatric medicine, and child and parent development—is less obscure and more easily understood. The glossary below is an attempt to (1) take the mystery out of the language of pediatrics and (2) to respect the intellect of parents. After years of experience I have little doubt that parents can understand pediatrics when it is explained, for they feel and live the experiences of pregnancy, childbirth, and child and parent development firsthand.

AIRPLANE, THE: One of the most (if not the most) successful calming techniques discovered by parents is "The Airplane." The infant is held stomach side down on the parent's forearm, like holding a football. The parent's hand is supporting the infant's body by holding the diaper at the crotch. The infant's head is on the outside of the parent's elbow. The infant's arm and leg on one side are held between the parent's arm and trunk. The other arm and leg dangle free on the outside of the parent's forearm. See Book I for photos and more on this calming technique.

ANECDOTE: According to Webster's New International Dictionary, an anecdote is "a short narrative of an interesting, amusing, or curious incident often biographical and generally characterized by human interest." That's a perfect description of my use of anecdotes.

AREOLA: The darker-and-rougher-than-skin area surrounding the nipple between the skin of the breast and the nipple itself.

ATTACHMENT, BONDING: The process whereby in his first year of life, the infant forms an irreversibly intimate relationship with his parents and recognizes them as his and recognizes others as strangers or nonparents. The importance of its necessity and strength cannot be overestimated; it is critical for the child's security, and later in his own life of intimacy. It is an extraordinarily complex process with even a biochemical nature to it. It takes place even in adoption. The process is not as fragile as first thought, and minor events that may interfere with closeness will not interfere with eventual successful bonding.

BIRTH PLAN: This is a well thought out, written plan that includes whom you want for a birthing coach, who is present in the room for support, how you want to manage pain, and other comparable matters. Written usually with your birth professional and presented to all involved, it expresses your wishes for delivery. Some are also recommending a second "Skills-based Birth Plan." These plans typically outline what you feel you can do given what skills you have learned that will augment your delivery. Programs that teach birthing skills include, for example, the Lamaze Method, the Bradley Method, Hypno-birthing, Hypno-babies, and Birthing Better.

BONDING: See ATTACHMENT, BONDING above.

CIRCADIAN: Noting or pertaining to rhythmic biological cycles, usually of sleep, recurring at approximately 24-hour intervals.

COLIC (adjective: COLICKY): Episodes of seemingly severe, acute abdominal pain in the very small infant. Infants experiencing colic double up while squirming and crying. Usually colic is simply abdominal discomfort in an infant with the "high strung," hypersensitive temperament. But there are other causes, such as GER (see "Gastroesophageal reflux"), and it may take a bit of detective work and patience to determine the root cause. Most colic comes on around three weeks of age and disappears by three-and-a-half months of age.

CUDDLER: A cuddly infant.

DOULA: Also known as a labor coach and originating from the Ancient

Greek word δούλη (meaning "female servant or slave"), a doula is a nonmedical person who assists a woman before, during, and after childbirth, as well as her partner and/or family by providing information, physical assistance, and emotional support. To find a doula visit www.dona.org.

FETUS (adjective: FETAL): After an ovum is fertilized by a sperm the fertilized ovum (or embryo) attaches to the wall of the uterus and grows. After the first three months or so the growing fertilized egg is termed a fetus.

GASTROESOPHAGEAL REFLUX (GER): This is a condition wherein the valve between the esophagus (the food tube between the mouth and the stomach) and the stomach does not function properly. Thus, milk does not stay in the stomach but refluxes back up the esophagus. The regurgitated stomach acid then irritates the esophagus and causes pain. If the GER is sufficiently severe, the ingested food is vomited back up and the infant fails to obtain adequate nutrition and weight gain. If the regurgitated milk goes up the esophagus but then down the respiratory track, the infant can have difficulty breathing. Parents do not need to worry if there is normal spit-up without pain, without respiratory problems, and there is normal weight gain.

GASTROCOLIC REFLEX: When food hits the stomach, not only does the stomach start to process it but the entire intestinal tract is also activated. Consequently, if stool or gas is in the lower large intestine, the infant has an urge to pass it. Thus, in the newborn period, it is not uncommon for a high-strung infant to start feeding and, less than a minute later arch his back and cry because of a gaseous cramp. He may then even pass stool (and often does).

GRADING SYSTEM: In the rite of passage of delivering a baby and raising a child, parents will grade themselves on how well they perceive themselves to be doing their job. Others, including friends, relatives, and practical strangers, may grade them as well. See the Index of Book I for an extensive discussion.

GUILT: This is the feeling we have if we feel responsible for something that has gone wrong, or is not proper. We feel it is our fault, or we could have prevented it, or made it better. There are many, many times when parents feel a preoccupation with the correctness of their actions as parents. Guilt is often not rational. The origins for this irrational feeling are twofold: (1) There is an egocentric quality to guilt: Guilt makes me important and implies the ability to be able to control everything. It is my fault! (2) Guilt is also a magical way of punishing oneself without having to change the presumably incorrect behavior. Guilt is not simply worry or concern.

GUILTEE: The author's neologism referring to the person being "guilted" in the "guilting" process.

GUILTER: Another of the author's neologisms referring to the one who, for a variety of reasons, dumps guilt on another, that is, the "guiltee."

GUILTING: Guilting is the act or acts of making another feel guilty. Guilt here is used as a verb rather than a noun.

"HIGH-STRUNG" TEMPERAMENT: An infant with this type of temperament is dominated by his newborn reflexes. His high sensitivity to touch and loud noises easily evokes his Moro startle reflex. His inability to control these reflexes is extraordinarily frustrating for him; and he expresses his frustration with a piercing, angry scream. He is frustration-intolerant unlike his opposite, the infant with a "laid-back" temperament. While initially challenging, the high-strung infant will likely become quite delightful with time and nurturing.

HOMEOSTASIS: Inherent in the "mothering role," homeostasis is the wish to have things calm and quiet, everything in its right place, and the maintenance of order and stability. It is the maternal role's drive for the status quo in the environment and in the child. Homeostasis is sought for both the happiness of the child and the parent; it is necessary for the coping of the mother. Its confronting opposite is the Kamikaze mode of the fathering role. Parental "roles," while gender-related, are not gender-specific.

HOMEOSTATIC PERIOD OF DEVELOPMENT: This period takes place around three-and-a-half months of age when the task of the infant is to calm himself and to work for dominance over the unsettling newborn reflexes that make purposeful movements so difficult. He may then begin to master control, calm himself, and perform many more intentional behavioral tasks. Prior to this time the infant, particularly the "high-strung" infant, is unable to calm himself.

HOMUNCULUS PHENOMENON: Parents may react toward or treat the infant regardless of age as if he were a homunculus, or a miniature adult.

HYPERSENSITIVE, HYPERREFLEXIVE: See REFLEX-DOMINATED NEWBORN and HIGH-STRUNG NEWBORN.

INDIVIDUATION: This is a terribly important process in the psychological development of children and adults from birth to death. A person, whether infant, child, or adult, gradually realizes that he/she is an individual. That conceptualization means understanding the power of independency and the consequences of being alone in that independency (that is, needing others as dependency).

Obviously, at times we are more powerful. At other times, such as when we are either very young or very old, we are more dependent. At each stage the infant—or later the child, adolescent, or adult—becomes more separate and independent.

The first individuation process occurs at about 18 months. The second individuation process is during pre-puberty, and puberty. The third individuation process involves leaving the home, as hallmarked for many by going to college. Then, aside from marriage (which is a separation-individuation ritual), I believe the next true individuation occurs just after thirty years of age when we realize our limits and that we are vulnerable and will not live forever. We continue to achieve and aspire until middle age when we must accept another individuation or reevaluation of our concept of ourselves. This is the gist of the book *Passages* by Gail Sheehy.

Perhaps the most interesting is the final individuation process, often seen in old age. The elderly often do not care what anyone else thinks about them or their behavior. They feel free and entitled to be and behave exactly as they feel, often regardless of others and others' feelings.

INTIMACY DRIVE: In healthy environments, both parents and the newborn infant are literally driven to recognize each other, become close, and evolve toward an intimate relationship. Sensuality is initially the most significant means by which this instinctually driven desire is accomplished. The parents snuggle, caress, and seek eye contact. The infant eventually responds and, when physically capable, dives back into the parents' bodies. This is one of the most powerful and wonderful drives of all animals, including humans.

The closeness of the intimacy drive in an infant imprints for his intimate relationships later in life. As he separates he seeks intimate relationships with others. He seeks close friends. He tries out partners and eventually chooses a spouse for the development of a deeper intimacy. The Intimacy Drive has now gone full circle.

Along the way mentors are found. The young adult develops intimate, trusting relationships to reach certain aspirations.

INTRUDER COMPLEX: The mixture of feelings in which parents consciously or unconsciously sense the reality of their new infant's intrusion into their own, the parents', life of intimacy together. These feelings begin during the pregnancy and persist throughout each child's development, and thereafter.

IN UTERO: A Latin phrase meaning within the uterus. An example would be to say that the baby is developing beautifully *in utero.*

IQ: Intelligence Quotient is a measure of intelligence obtained from standardized tests of children and adults. The average is 100.

JAUNDICE: Newborns often have some degree of jaundice. It comes about as follows: Red blood cells carry oxygen from the lungs to the body tissues and take carbon dioxide back to the lungs to be exhaled. Red blood cells are like skin or hair; they have a life cycle. In the newborn, they live about 100 days; some are being born and some are dying off all the time. When they die off, they burst open and the red-pigmented hemoglobin inside pops out. An enzyme that opens it up immediately nicks it and changes the way light shines through it. It is no longer red, but now is yellow. That is jaundice. It is a yellow pigment in the skin and the whites of the eyes. The liver then sees the buildup and turns on, usually around day three. It then processes the bilirubin (jaundice).

KAMIKAZE MODE: A father will often interact with the infant in a way that adventurously appears disruptive (or Kamikaze) of the usual routine established by the mother. It prepares the child for the aspects of life that are chaotic or competitive. It counterbalances the homeostasis, which a mother desires and establishes. Dr. James Herzog first described the Kamikaze Mode in fathers in 1977.

LAMAZE [birthing] METHOD: In 1951 in France, Dr. Fernand Lamaze introduced his method whereby mothers and fathers went through pregnancy and childbirth together after experiencing education classes on relaxation and breathing techniques from a specially trained nurse. The Lamaze methods took hold and grew tremendously following their introduction to the United States in the 1960s. Courses/classes are now available almost everywhere.

LETDOWN REFLEX (Also known now as the milk ejection reflex): When a breast-feeding infant first attaches to the nipple, a stimulus goes through the mother's nerves up the spinal cord and to the brain, initiating the secretion of two hormones into the blood stream from the pituitary gland at the base of the brain. One of the hormones tells the breasts to make milk. The other literally pumps the milk out. That is the so-called let down reflex, as the milk comes out. A small microscopic cuff of smooth muscle tissue is present around every duct in the breast. When the hormone hits the muscle, it contracts and milks the milk out. That hormone also acts on another smooth muscle, namely the muscle of the uterus. It is not at all uncommon for breast-feeding mothers to complain of uterine cramps or increased blood flow with nursing in the immediate postpartum period. This also helps the uterus to return to its pre-pregnancy size.

MENTOR: A mentor is a close, trusted, and experienced counselor or guide. To me, a mentor is a trusted person who bridges the gap between being dependent upon one's parents and being fully independent.

MIDWIFE: A woman in Western societies who is skilled in delivering babies from low-risk pregnancies. In third world countries obstetricians, nurse practitioners, and skilled midwifes are hard to find, so midwifes are used always for deliveries; many are quite skilled and experienced.

MILK EJECTION REFLEX: See the LETDOWN REFLEX.

MORO STARTLE REFLEX: The startle reflex of the newborn in which they look as if they are falling. Their arms fling out in an arched embrace and they have a frightened, startled, wide-eyed expression. Newborns do this when tossed into the air or placed on their backs. They do not do it when placed on their stomachs because their arms are secure.

NARCISSITIC REJECTION: In the Greek myth, Narcissus was condemned by an avenging goddess to hopelessly fall in love with his own image reflecting back to him from a crystal-clear fountain. All of us appreciate, narcissistically, aspects of ourselves and often like to think that the positive qualities of our offspring belong to us and to our side of the family. To that end, we imagine any negative qualities in our offspring come from somewhere else, in most cases the other side of the family. That is known as narcissistic rejection.

NEOLOGISM: A new word not found in any dictionary that, in this case, is coined by the author for its graphic explanatory effect.

NEONATE: Another word for newborn. A neonatal intensive care unit is an intensive care unit for newborns.

NURSE PRACTITIONERS: Nurses who have advanced, postgraduate training (for example, in obstetrics). Nurse practitioners assume some of the duties that were formally limited to just physicians, like delivering babies from normal, low-risk pregnancies. They are often required to have an obstetrician backup available. There are also Pediatric Nurse Practitioners.

OBSTETRICIAN (OB): A doctor who is certified to deliver babies and manages all the complications related to delivery.

OVUM: An unfertilized egg.

PARENT TERMINOLOGY: m/f stands for a mother/father dyad, m/m for mother/mother, f/f for father/father parents (m is not for male and f is not for female in this book series).

PEDIATRICIAN: A doctor who is trained and certified to handle health problems of young patients, ranging from birth through college or so.

POSTPARTUM: A medical phrase referring to the span of time just after delivery of a baby.

PROJECTION: See GUILT and GUILTING. To protect oneself from feeling guilty, it is less painful to blame someone else. We project the guilt onto them and off ourselves. We can also then be angry with the object of our projection because it is now their fault; we are no longer fearful that it is our fault. A common expression of projected guilt is real anger (based in fear), which is usually less painful to bear than real self-guilt.

POSTTRAUMATIC STRESS DISORDER (PTSD): A mental condition in which a previous trauma in one's life is relived in flashbacks that interfere with one's emotional or work life or that become debilitating. These flashbacks can come as nightmares but can be and more commonly are memories with a visceral, or gut-wrenching, feeling.

RAPPROCHEMENT: In terms of child development, rapprochement is the period between the independent pride of the newly accomplished toddler and the toilet-trained, two- to three-year-old child. It is the period when the toddler, now beyond his ecstatic accomplishment of walking, has suddenly realized his locomotion has placed distance between himself and his parents. He neither wants to lose his newfound independence nor the security of his mother and father. It is a time of built-in pride and also unhappiness. The child is torn between secure dependency and the thrill of independence.

REFLEX-DOMINATED NEWBORN: The particular type of temperament of a newborn child who is (1) dominated by the newborn reflexes, (2) sensitive to stimuli that set off these reflexes, and (3) vehemently expresses his frustration over his lack of control over these reflexes. Years ago, this type of newborn was termed the "hypertonic" newborn. Others have also called him the "jittery" newborn.

REFUELING: Refueling occurs in the rapprochement phase when the locomoting toddler toddles away and separates himself from his mother or father but returns to grasp and hug her/his legs to seek reassurance. He "refuels" or endeavors to obtain further reassuring energy to go away from the parent again in an ever-widening circle. He wants the guarantee that he has not and will not lose his mother/father in his adventures.

REGRESSION: The act or process of behaving much younger than one's actual chronological age, that is, behaving "like a baby."

"RESCUE vs. EMPATHY": These are the two alternative methods of coping with an infant or child's frustrations and problems. "Rescue" indicates that the parent saves the child from the frustration by solving the problem for him instead of giving a child a chance to master the difficulty himself. Empathy entails temporarily identifying with the child, feeling his feelings of frustration, and supportively and lovingly encouraging the infant/child to self-mastery. Empathy permits the infant/child to resolve the dilemma. With empathy, the parent does not abandon the child but stays with and supports him with warm understanding while allowing him to conquer the problem. Newborns need close to 100 percent rescue, while twenty-something-year-old offspring need close to 100 percent empathy. Over the days, weeks, months, and years that their children grow, parents must learn to swing the pendulum slowly from rescue to empathy.

RITES OF PASSAGE: Ethnographer Arnold van Gennep in 1909 first described these Rites of Passage as involving age-old, often centuries-old rituals that help all the different members of a culture or group adjust to the change of the individual(s) as he/she separates from one group to join (or intrude into) another. The ritual validates the change and helps all accept the loss/separation from the first group and intrusion into the new group. Examples are Bris, Baptism, Bar and Bat Mitzvah, Graduations, Marriage, and Birthing. See SEPARATION RITUALS.

SEPARATION: The child becomes conscious of being a separate little person and, in developing, learns to separate himself from his parents. The attachment is not lost even though there is separation in time, space, and from the symbiotic aspects of the attachment.

SEPARATION FEARS: When a child is around 4-and-a-half months of age, he becomes smarter, and for the first time becomes aware of being separate from the mother. With that awareness comes a fear: "*If I am separate, I can be separated, I can be alone!*" The fear shows up initially in two ways: The first is stranger anxiety, which occurs when a child becomes anxious as he realizes that he can be separated from his mother or father by, for example, an exuberant relative who wants to hold and hug him. The second is night waking. With the realization of separateness, an infant wakes up and fearfully wonders where his parents are. He cries out with fear, which is often misunderstood by the parents as hunger or teething. These fears are actually a good problem because they are a manifestation of the close attachment to the parents, particularly the symbiotic attachment with the mother. It is especially gratifying to see these feelings in an adopted child. The task in front of the child is to learn to trust that he will not be abandoned. Separation fears continue throughout all of development and are felt by parents as well. While parents are happy to see a child grow and develop, there is a sadness. It is felt as the infant with growth and development matures towards more and more independence eventually emerging in adulthood.

SEPARATION-INDIVIDUATION: See INDIVIDUATION; SEPARATION.

SEPARATION RITUALS: Separation rituals that celebrate the child's separate existence from his parents exist in all cultures. They are usually informal ceremonies sanctioning the separation of the child from the parents, particularly from the mother from whose womb he was initially inseparable. Examples include naming ceremonies, the Navajo "laughing" ceremony, the first haircut (particularly for Hindus), going to nursery school, ear piercing, confirmations and bar mitzvahs, leaving for college, getting married, and having a child. These rituals are also called "rites of passage."

SIBLING RIVALRY: When a newborn arrives (or even prior to arrival) an older brother or sister will resent having to share his parents with the new baby. This rivalry with the baby for the mother can be seen by attention-getting behavior such as regressive or younger behavior (wetting or soiling, and/or overt physical aggression toward the younger sibling). As the younger child grows, he too may compete with his sibling for his mother's attention.

SINE QUA NON: A Latin phrase for something indispensable, that without which nothing else would exist or occur.

SOCERAPHOBIA: The fear of in-laws

SONOGRAM: Sound waves are sent toward and bounced off a structure, and the recording equipment monitors the changed bounced-backed returning waves. The reflected waves' measurements can be put together to form an image of the structure and this image can be monitored on a television screen. This is a sonogram. Sonograms are safely and commonly used to obtain a picture of the fetus in the womb. Sonography can also be used to harmlessly look at the heart and other organs. When looking at the heart, it is called an echocardiogram.

SPERM: The motile male reproductive cell produced by the testes that comes out of the penis in the semen during orgasm. When introduced within the vagina, sperm travel up through the uterus seeking an ovum. When a sperm finds the ovum, it plunges inside the ovum and fertilizes it.

STARTLE REFLEX: See MORO STARTLE REFLEX.

STILLBORN: A birth in the final months of pregnancy or at the end of pregnancy of a baby who is not alive.

STOOL: Feces, or the material passed out the anus during the defecation process.

STRANGER ANXIETY: An infant often expresses stranger anxiety, one of the worries of separation fears, as early as four-and-a-half months of age. See SEPARATION FEARS.

SUDDEN INFANT DEATH SYNDROME (SIDS): Is the unexplained death, usually during sleep, of a seemingly healthy baby less than a year old. Sometimes called "crib death." Fortunately, SIDS is rare; but it is frequently talked about by parents and experts. Studies show that SIDS is largely preventable, albeit not completely so, by having the infant sleep on his back instead of his side or stomach. It occurs more often in winter, more often with lots of blankets and stuffed animals in the crib, more often if the infant is sleeping on his stomach, and more often between the ages of three to nine months.

SYMBIOTIC ATTACHMENT, SYMBIOSIS: The relationship usually between the mother and child whereby their feelings are often indistinguishable from each other. For example, when an infant receives an immunization shot, the mother often feels his discomfort; she may actually feel it to the extent that it is as if she were actually receiving the shot herself. To avoid this, some mothers will leave the room while the immunization is given. This symbiosis, or merge of feelings, is part of the basis for adult intimacy, empathy, and closeness.

TEMPERAMENT: The (probably) genetically determined disposition of an infant, child, or for that matter adult. Parents can develop a reasonably good idea of their infant's temperament soon after birth. The spectrum of temperament ranges from the quiet, cuddly, laid-back infant to the high-strung, hyper-reflexive, hypersensitive, frustration-intolerant newborn.

TENP: An acronym for Temperament Evaluation of the Newborn, an evaluation system developed by Dr. Paul Peebles. See Book I for details, process, and answers.

TERM: "Term" is the expression for the end of a normal pregnancy of nine months or forty weeks. "Preterm" indicates that the infant was born prior to the full forty-week term. Likewise, "postterm" indicates the newborn was born after the usual forty weeks of gestation.

TRANSITIONAL OBJECTS: Transitional objects are the child's symbols of attachment, much like we parents carry pictures of our children in our wallets. Transitional objects represent the mother, and/or father. They allow the child to make the transition from the close symbiotic attachment with the mother to being able to literally and figuratively "stand on his own two feet." Transitional objects fall into three categories: (1) oral objects (e.g., pacifiers, prolonged use of the bottle, and thumbs), (2) warm and cuddly things (e.g., teddy bears and blankets), or (3) the mother's and later the child's own hair.

TRICHOTILLOMANIA: This is the infatuation with holding and, later in adult life, twirling one's own hair when feeling the need to calm oneself. When separation fears set in, some infants will, while snuggling with the mother or father, reach up and hold the parent's hair as it dangles down. Later, when not in the parent's arms, they will hold their own hair in remembrance of the closeness with the parent. It is a calming technique. Sometimes, when angry at their parents, these one-and-a-half to three-year-old children will pull out their own hair. When remorse follows the initial anger, a child may eat the pulled-out hair he holds in his hand. Rarely, this can lead to intestinal obstruction by a "hairball" in the stomach; the hairball's medical name is trichobezoar.

A later childhood an adult pathological form of pulling out one's hair and/or eyebrows is also called trichotillomania. This older child and young adult trichotillomania is an obsessive-compulsive disorder.

TRIMESTER: A pregnancy runs nine months under normal circumstances. Each of the three three-month periods of those nine months is called a trimester.

USURPER PERCEPTION: In the United States, prior to the 1960s only doctors delivered babies and primarily in hospitals. Only doctors, nurses, and the mother-to-be were allowed in the hospital birthing room. Fathers were excluded from the event, newborns were sent to newborn nurseries, and mothers were sent off to wards. Fortunately, this is a concept of the past (but it is worth remembering its origin so as to understand the present concept of delivery as a rite of passage). In the 1960s, the methods of French Dr. Lamaze were introduced in this country. Trained nurses taught breathing and relaxation techniques, fathers were allowed to be present as coaches, and delivery became a family event. Parents took back their roles in this rite of passage. It was perceived previously that the medical profession had usurped the parents' roles in this rite of passage, delivering the newborn as if the mother were a mere conduit. Now parents are in charge. They go through courses, such as the Lamaze classes, and establish Birth Plans. The medical profession is there in support, particularly in risky situations, to use their knowledge in true service to parents-to-be. Hence, the Usurper Perception is no longer an issue for many parents-to-be. Now fathers are involved in the delivery, they often stay overnight in the hospital with wife and child, and "rooming in" is allowed, whereby the newborn can stay with the parents in their hospital room for as much time as the parents wish.

"WISH vs. REALITY": The ever-present conflict in parents in which the wish for the child or infant does not conform with the reality that the child lives with and presents to us.

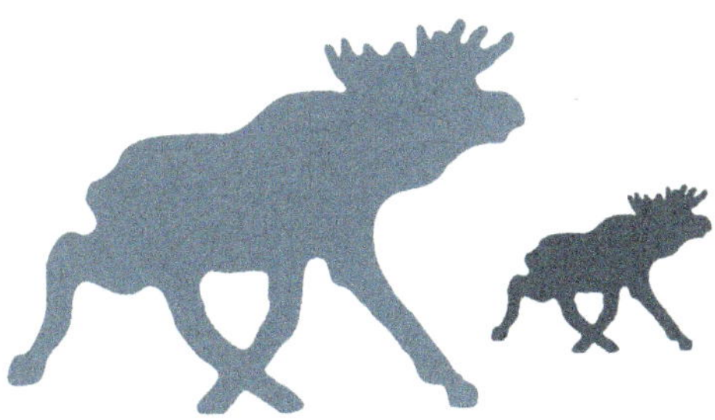

Index

K

L

M

N

O

P

R

S

T

U

V

W

Points Regarding Content and Investigation Methods

The points made in these books belong to and are garnered from many parents and their children, as well as our current pediatric knowledge and experience.

When I first went into practice, I felt ill-prepared to answer most questions that parents asked. Pediatricians are trained to handle heart failure and leukemia but very little training existed then for sleep problems and separation conflicts, and still very little is available in the literature regarding working with parents. Consequently, I met with small groups of parents to discuss all the issues that concerned them. It was from these small group discussions that the information and concepts in this series arose. Indeed, the parents and children have written this series. Certain concepts, like The Intruder Complex and its corollaries, have evolved from my personal observations and have been included only if seen in numerous situations and confirmed by many couples.

This book series arose from the observations of "normal" families, families without obvious pathology. Others have studied by observation normal child development, hence especially Mahler's separation-individuation research and Piaget's "object permanence," for example. Also, anthropological studies of normal families in different cultures have been described. But this series is more about the parents' interactions with each other and with themselves...and with their child, not about the development of the child alone.

I want to thank these families who have so generously shared their lives with me. I have made every effort to respect their confidentiality and identity. Consequently, while the themes in the stories told in these books are true, the names, dates, circumstances, and details are fictitious. Each story shared is supported by numerous similar situations that I have come across in my fifty years of experience. Indeed, most stories shared are conglomerates and the actors are amalgams. Any personal identification with any particular character is purely coincidental and related, more likely, to identification with the themes.

A few stories were so poignant that that I did not want to change them. Consequently, I received permission from the parents to relate these stories but have changed details so that the stories would not be recognizable by others. Some stories have been written by the parents themselves, and published with their permission.

Thank you, again, to all those families who shared their lives to help others.

Parents' Responsibilities

Several authorities have reviewed the information in this series for content and accuracy.

The content, which derives from the experience of many families over many years, is presented to serve as guidelines and not as absolutes for solving the numerous and various problems confronting today's parents. To individualize and solve a particular problem for a specific patient, parents must trust their own judgment and consult their own pediatrician. This series is not written with the intent to take the place of either the parent or pediatrician. If at any time parents feel that an infant has a serious illness, either physical or mental, he must be seen by a physician. The author and publisher thus cannot be held accountable for any problems or damaging effects resulting from any substitution of the thoughts and general guidelines of this book for the sound judgment of either parents and/or their doctors. Likewise, the author and publisher cannot be responsible for any misinterpretation or misapplication of any of the content in this book or its series.

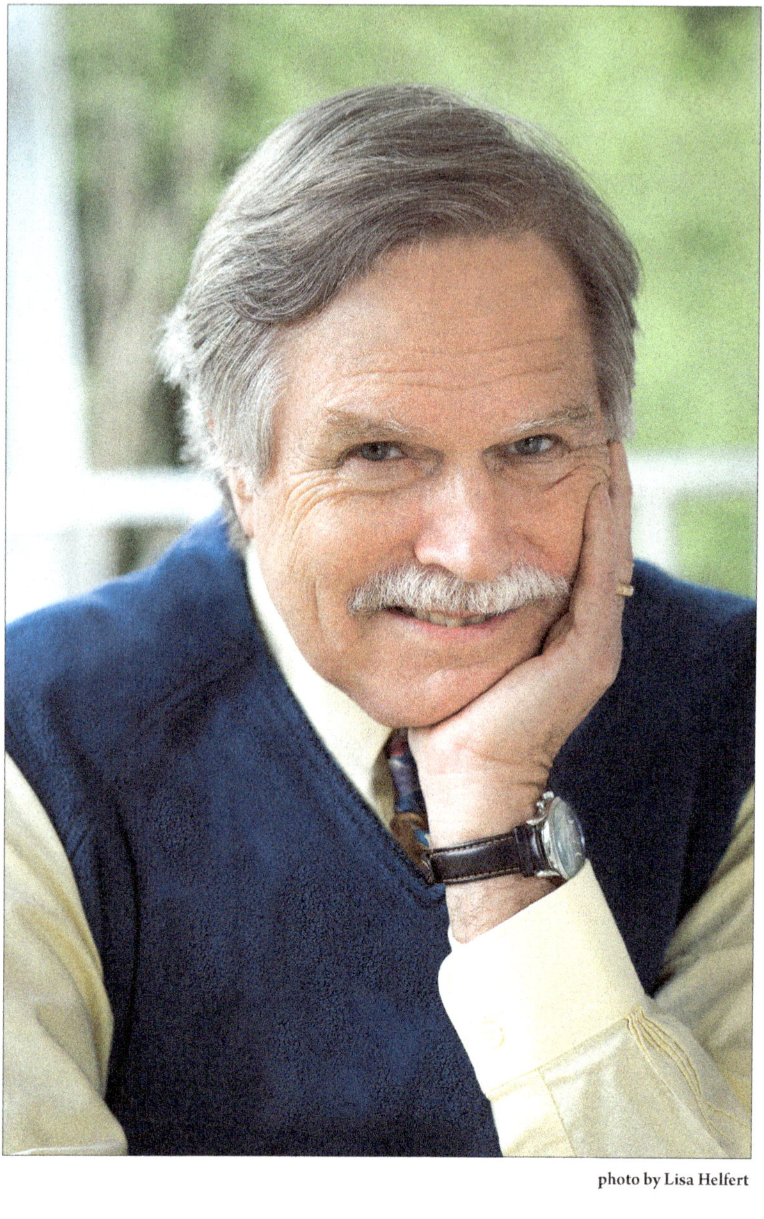

photo by Lisa Helfert

The Author

Paul Peebles, a husband, father of two, and grandfather of five, received his medical degree from Case Western Reserve University and completed his pediatric internship at University Hospitals (Cleveland) where his preceptor was Dr. Benjamin Spock. He fulfilled his residency at Harvard's Children's Hospital Medical Center (Boston) training with Dr. T. Berry Brazelton. He is Board Certified in both Pediatrics and Pediatric Hematology-Oncology with a special interest in Behavioral Pediatrics. Dr. Peebles served as a Clinical Associate, Staff Associate, and Senior Investigator at the National Institutes of Health (Washington, DC), and performed additional research at the Karolinska Institute (Stockholm) and at Children's Hospital Medical Center (Boston). He was on the faculties of Harvard University School of Medicine, the Johns Hopkins University School of Medicine (Baltimore), and Georgetown University's School of Medicine (Washington, DC). He is currently a Clinical Professor of Pediatrics at Children's National Medical Center of George Washington University's School of Medicine (Washington, DC). Dr. Peebles belongs to several professional societies, including the prestigious Society for Pediatric Research. He is currently in private practice as the founder and Director Emeritus of The Pediatric Care Center and Young Adult Care Center in Bethesda, Maryland. Dr. Peebles is a writer-scientist with many publications including articles with primary authorship published in *Nature* and *Science*. He commutes between Washington DC, Philadelphia, and Fiskebäckskil, Sweden. In *The Washingtonian* magazine, his peers have elected him as "one of the area's leading primary care physicians."

CPSIA information can be obtained
at www.ICGtesting.com
Printed in the USA
BVOW05s0026080617
486154BV00020B/150/P

9 780997 076233